DOT TO DOT BOOK FOR KIDS AGES 8-12

By Happy children

This book belong's to

_____

This book is for all the children of the world. Have a lot of fun.

Copyright © 2020 by Happy Children

ALL RIGHT RESERVED

No part of this book may be reproduced,stored in a retrieval system,or transmitted in any form or by any electronic,mechanical,photocopying,recording,scanning,or otherwise,without the prior written permission of the publisher.

To parents

Playing is a good time for a youngster, however it is additionally fundamental! Kids need to play to make disclosures, to comprehend their general surroundings and to foster well. Because of this playbook, they foster numerous abilities.
Spot to-dabs are an incredible fun, instructive exercise. Finishing a speck to-dab has numerous advantages:

Spot to-speck and then some

Chipping away at a dab to-spot trains kids number request and help with tallying. Little ones may require a little assistance, yet as they get more seasoned, finishing a speck to-spot without anyone else is an incredible certainty promoter.

Hand-eye co-appointment

Spot to-speck games are awesome for improving hand-eye co-appointment. There's a ton of focus that goes into finishing a spot to-dab! Visual engine control is created through speck to-spot work.

Penmanship abilities

Doing dab to-speck exercises truly improves penmanship abilities and are an important pre-composing instructing device. Youngsters figure out how to make shapes, center their pencil and figure out how much strain to apply to the paper.

Fine engine abilities

Dealing with a speck to-spot is an incredible method to reinforce hand and finger muscles in anticipation of composing. During youth is the ideal
 opportunity to help foster essential muscles we'll use for the duration of our life. Kids can focus on grasping their pencil and reinforce their hands while chipping away at spot to-speck.

let's go!

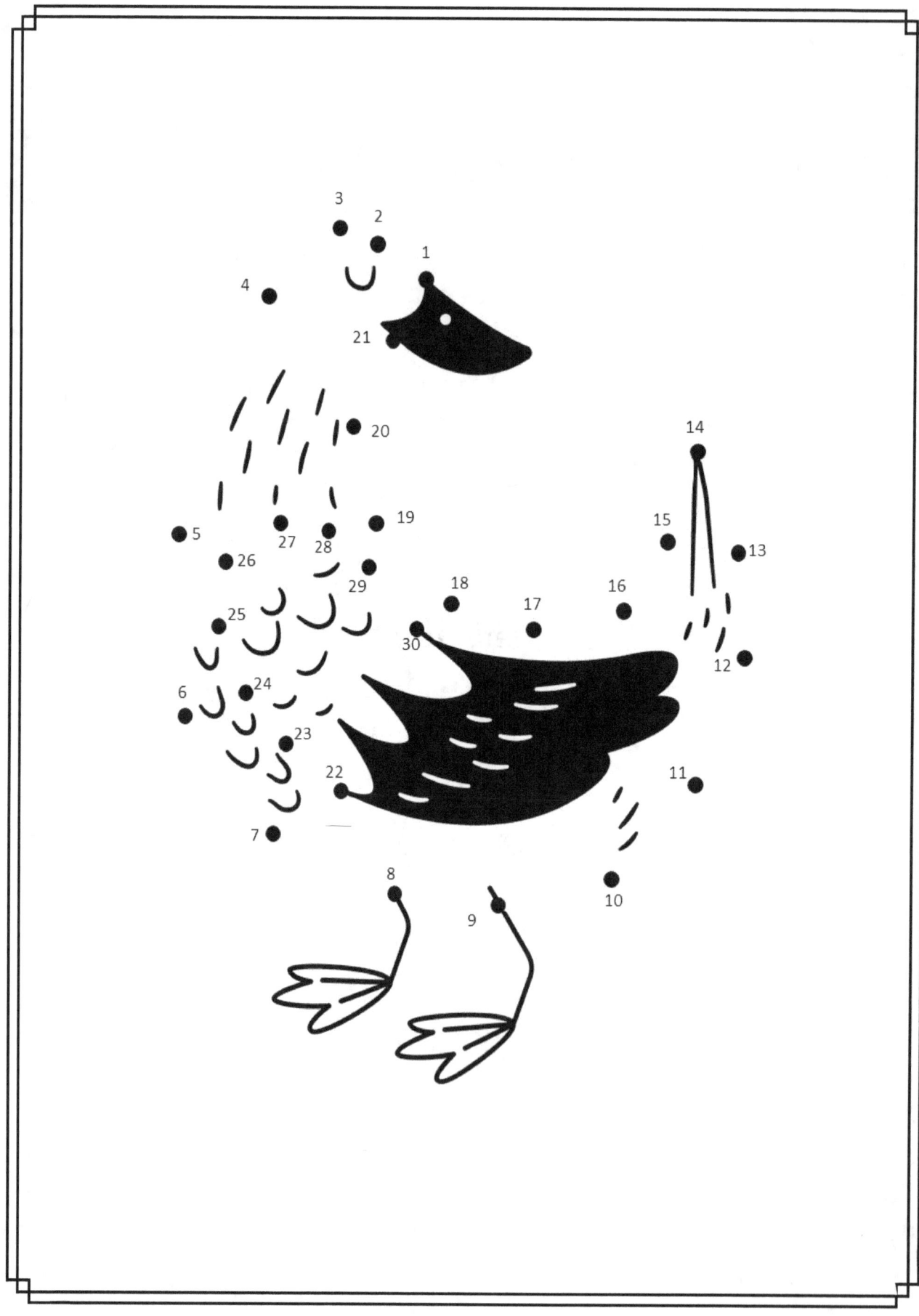

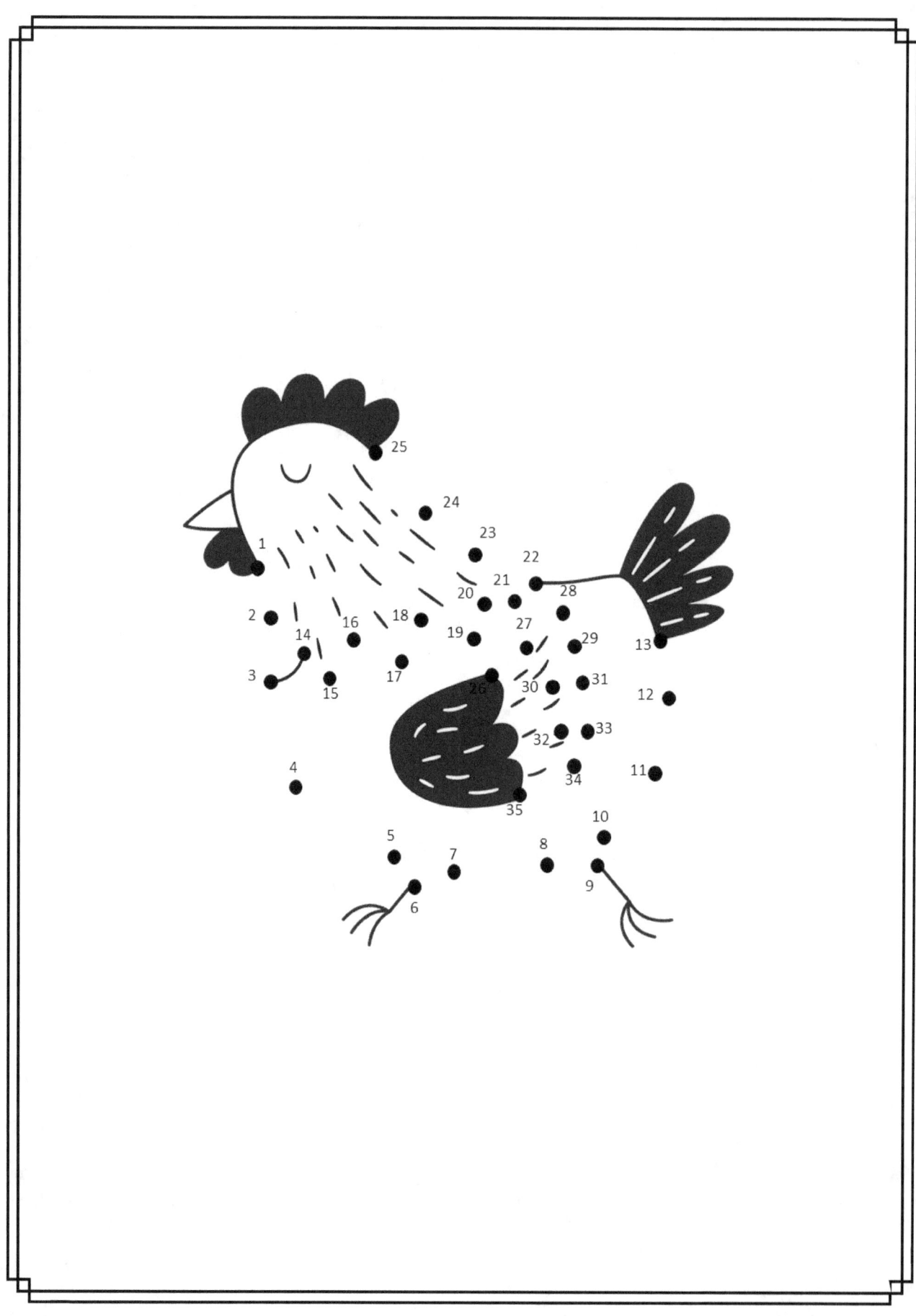

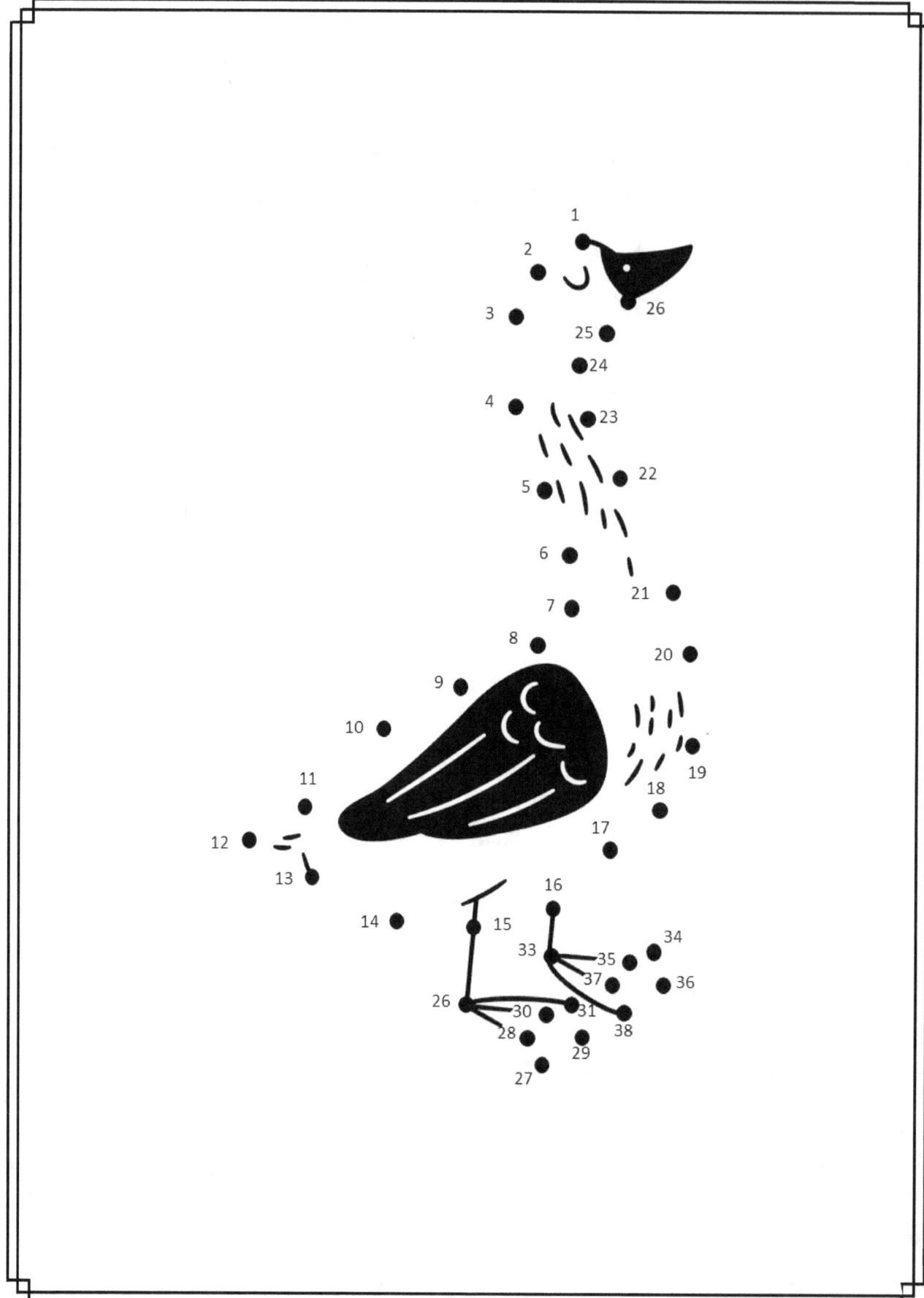

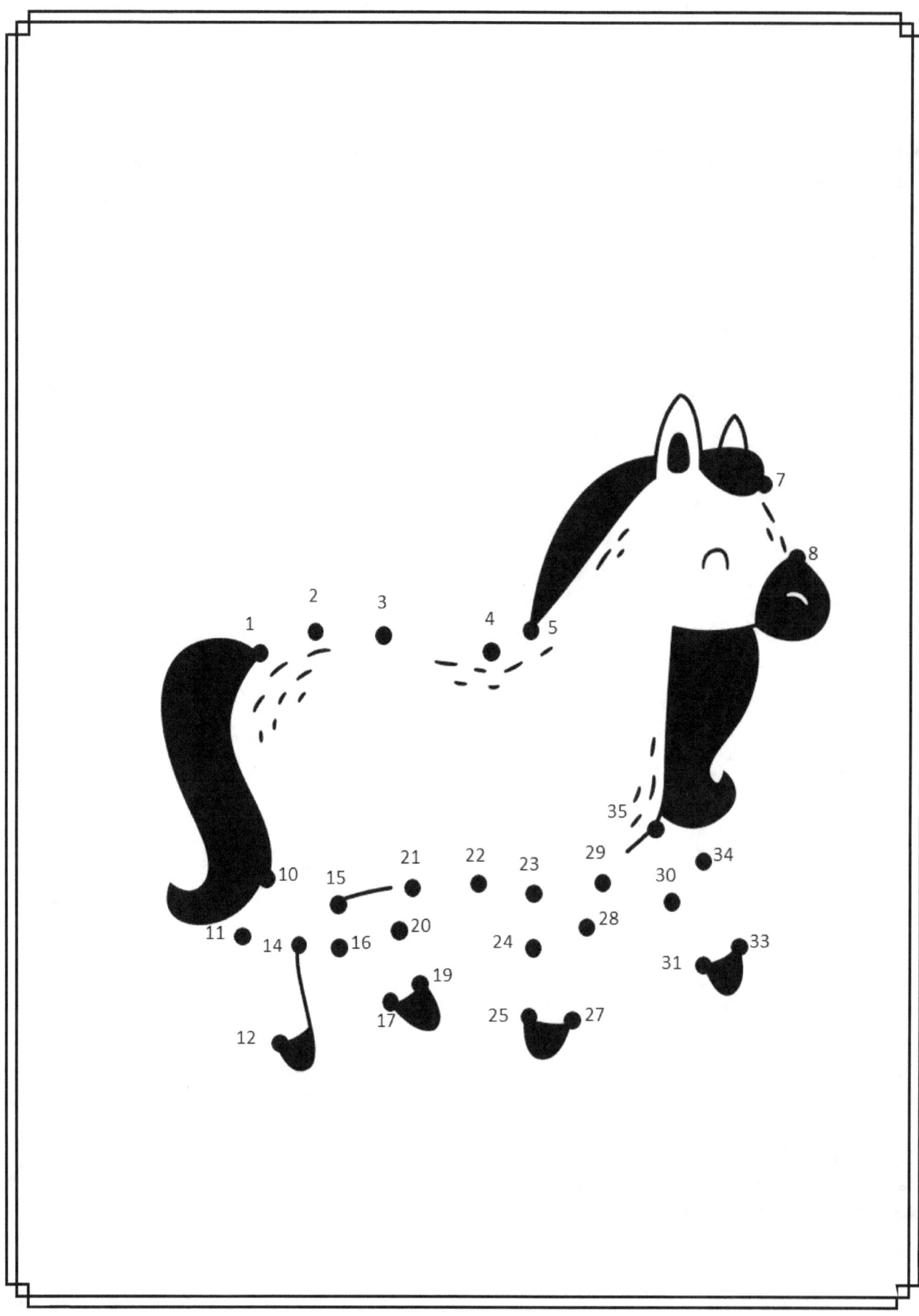

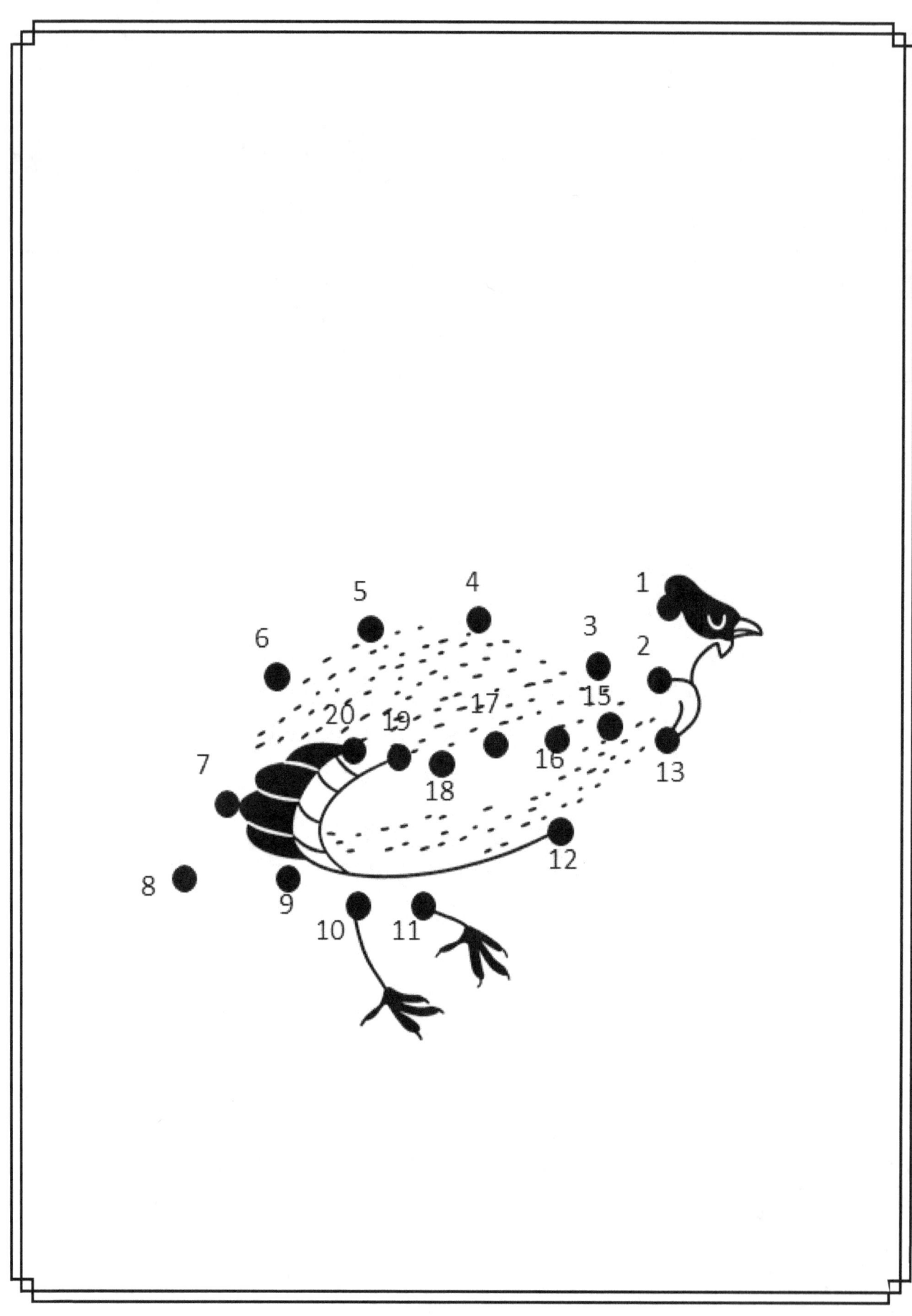

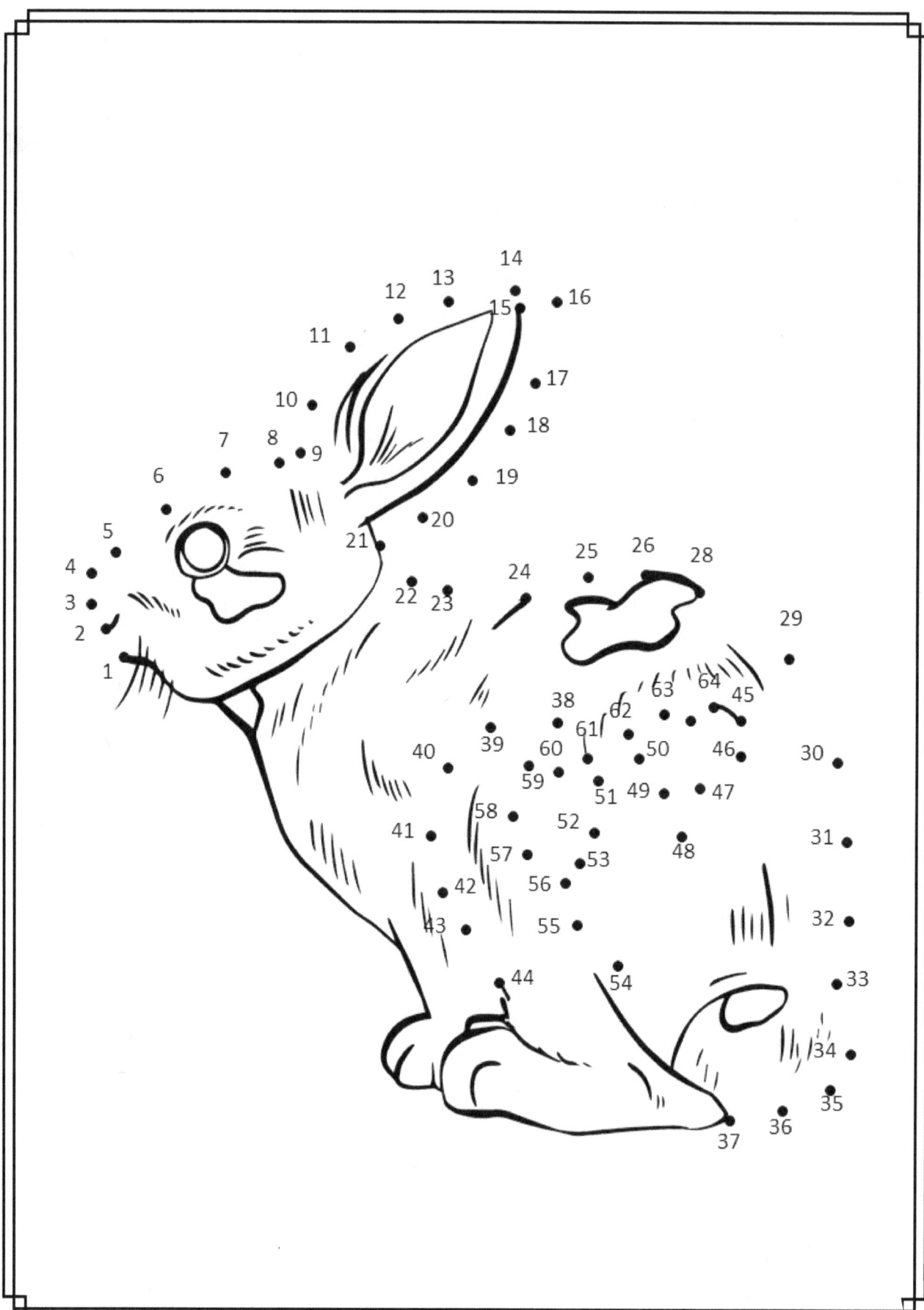

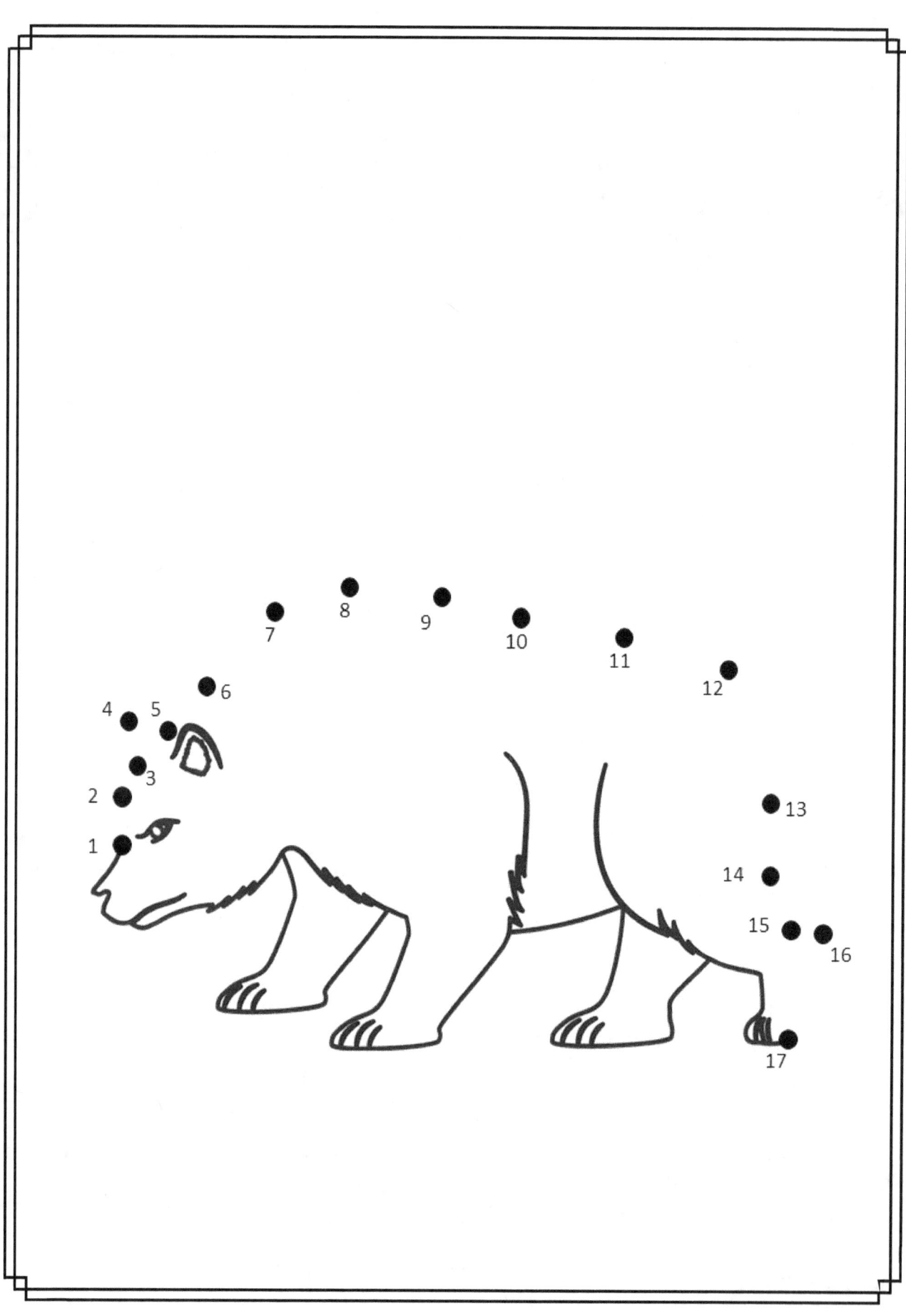

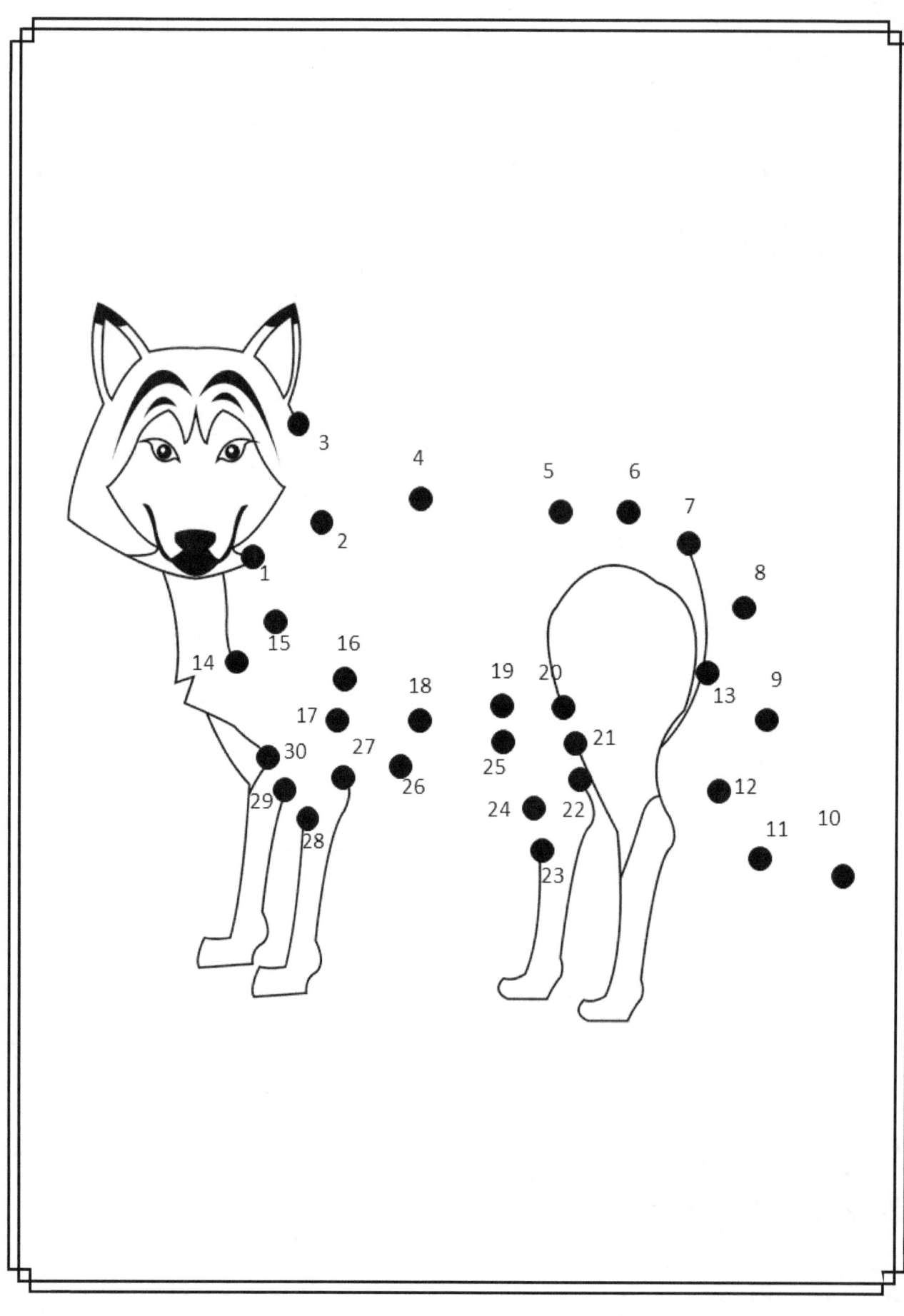

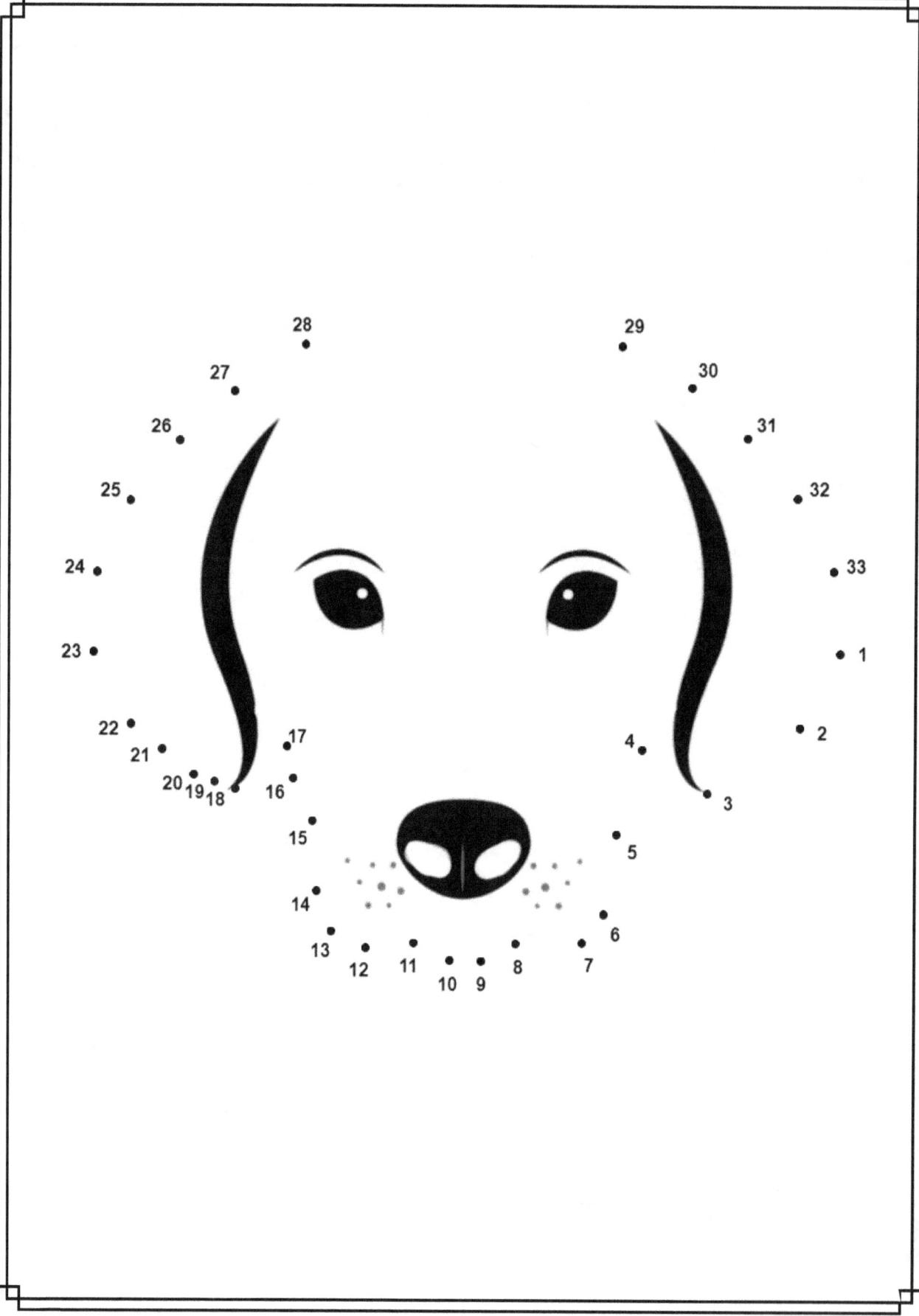

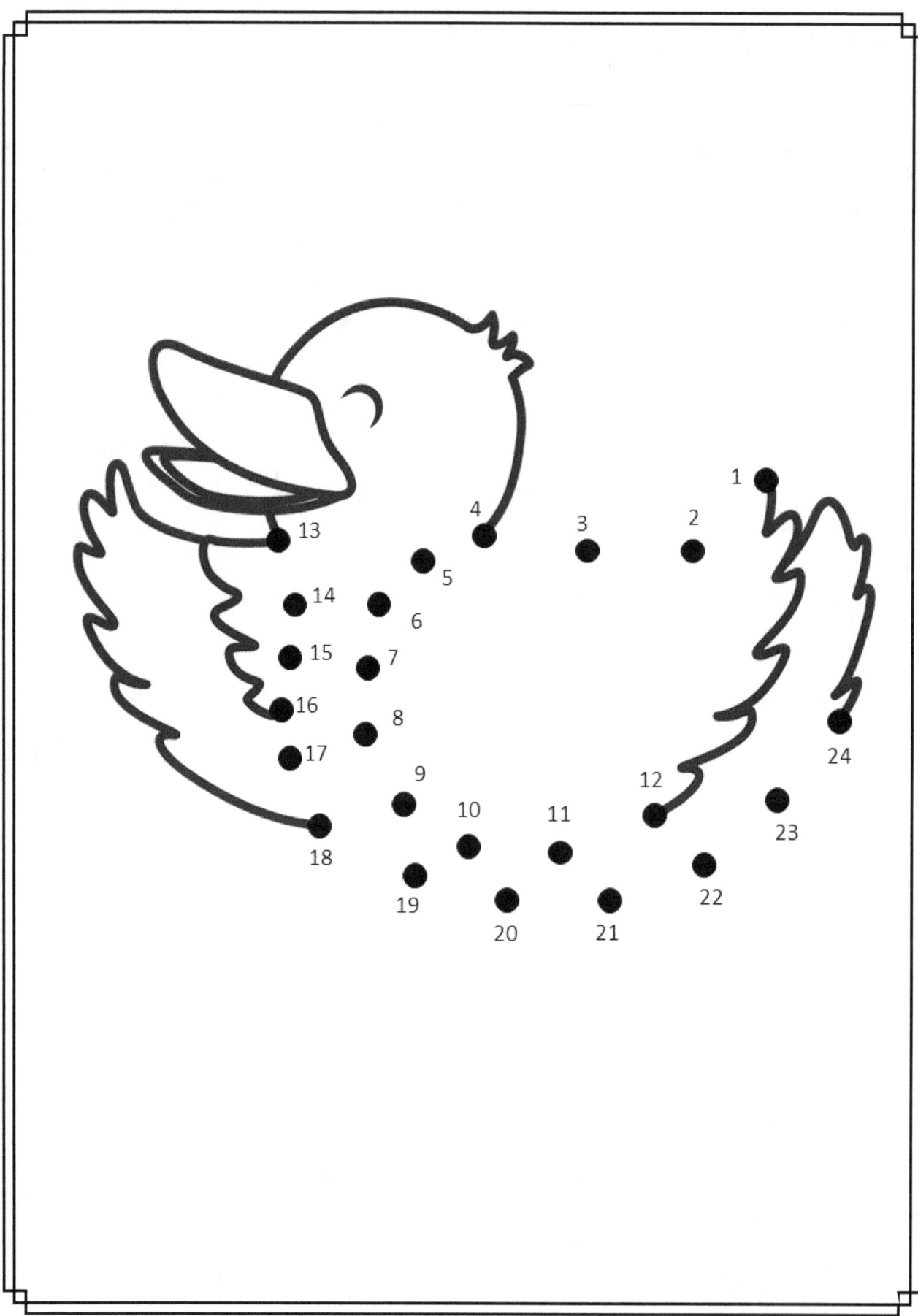

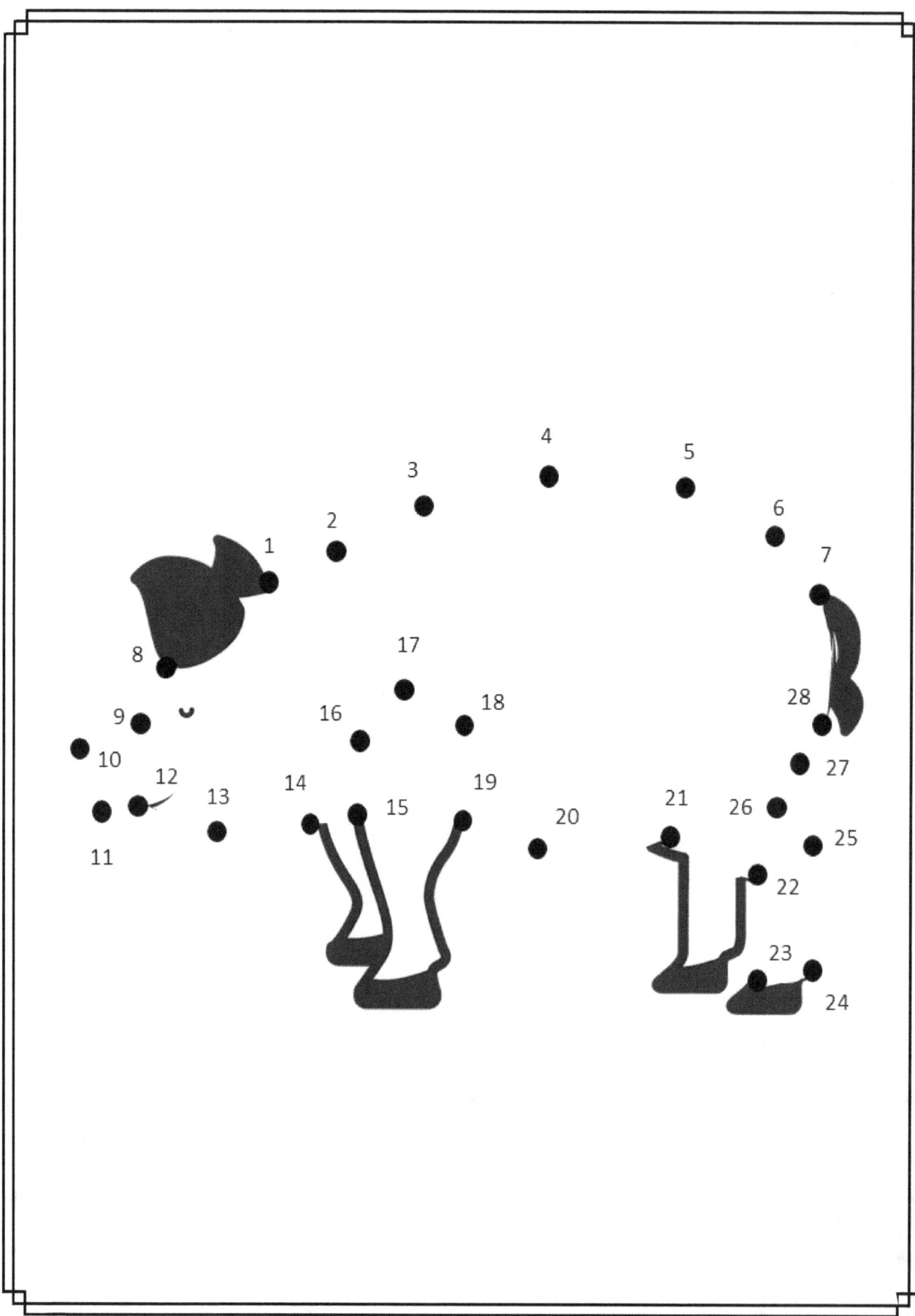

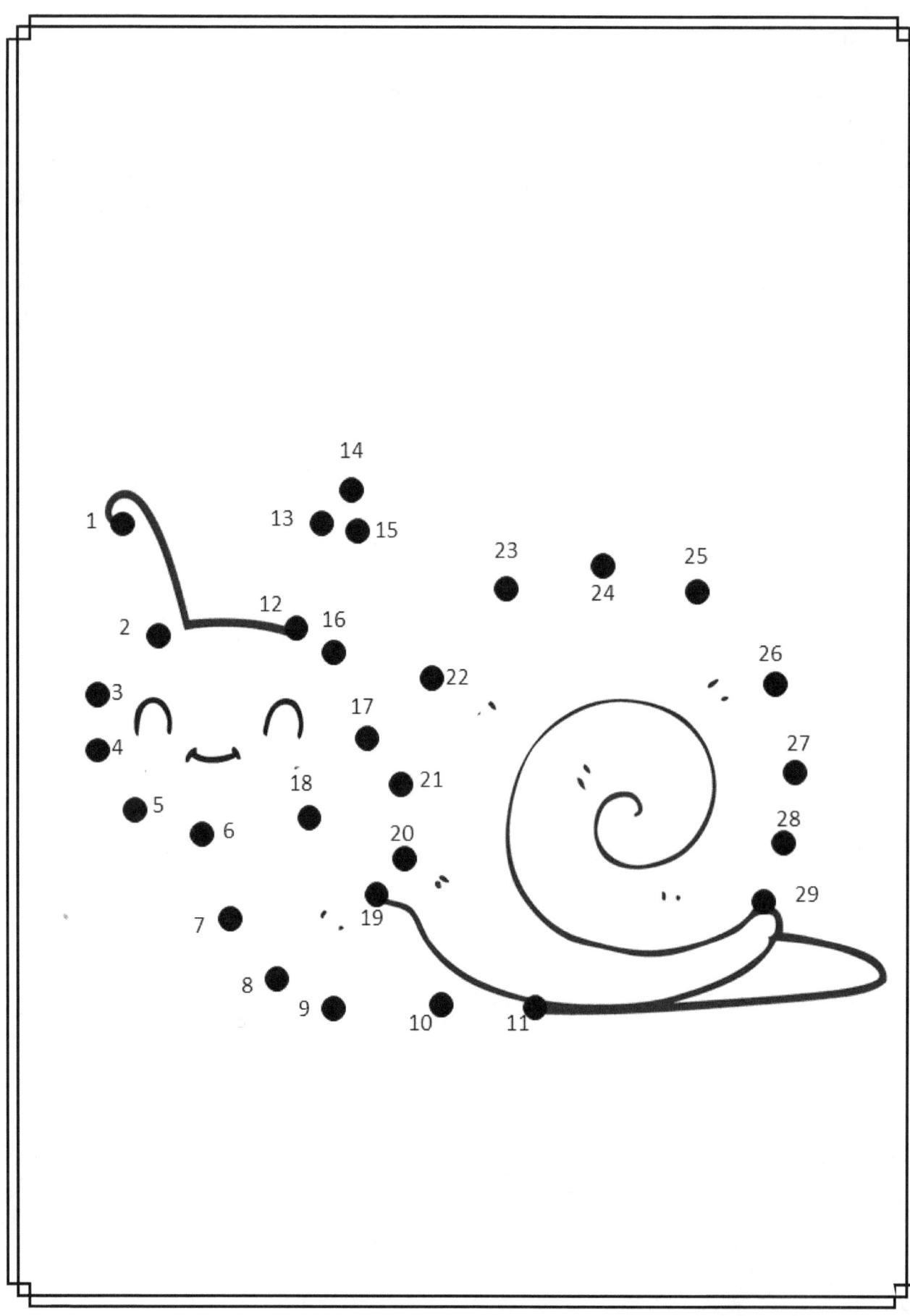

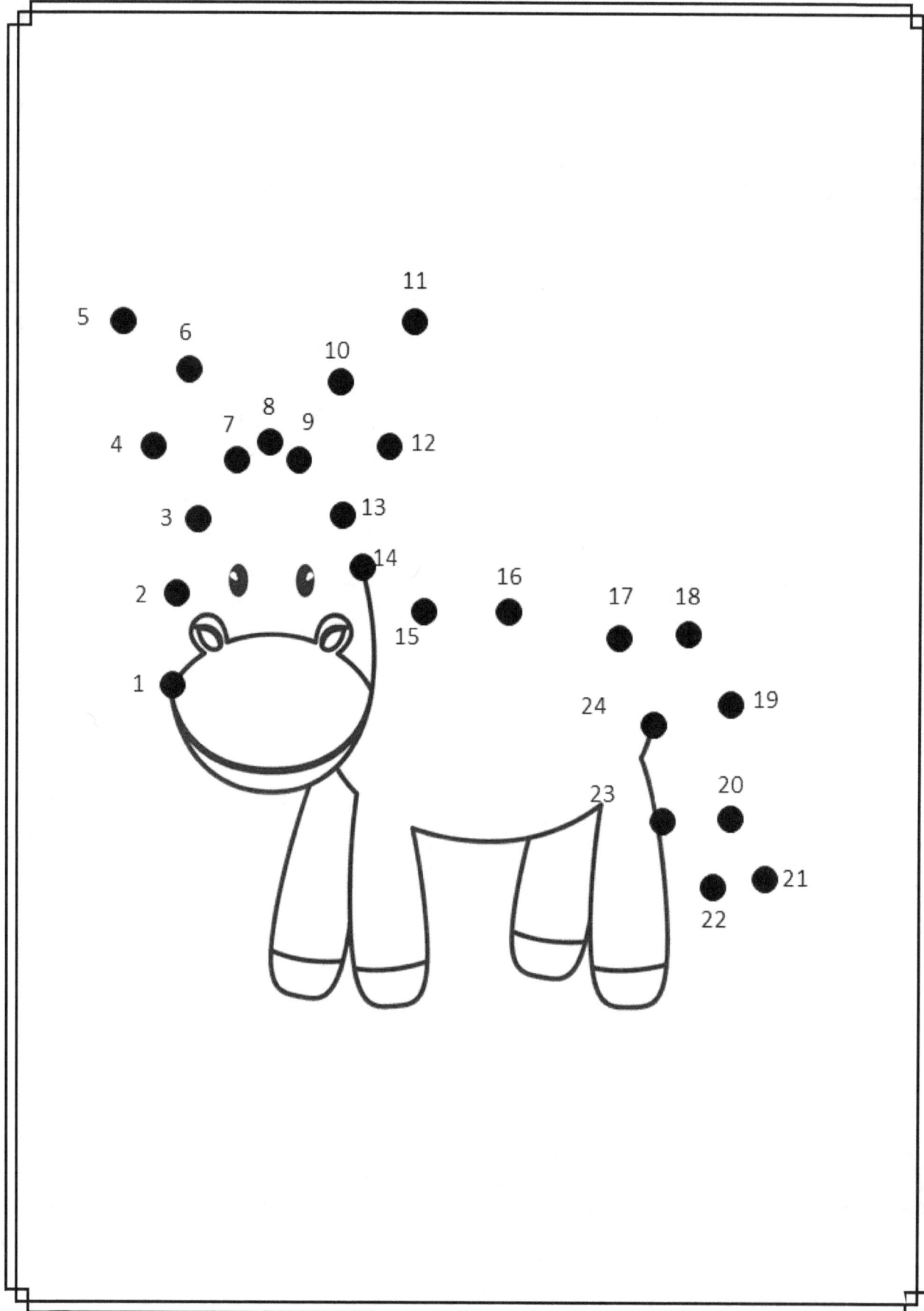

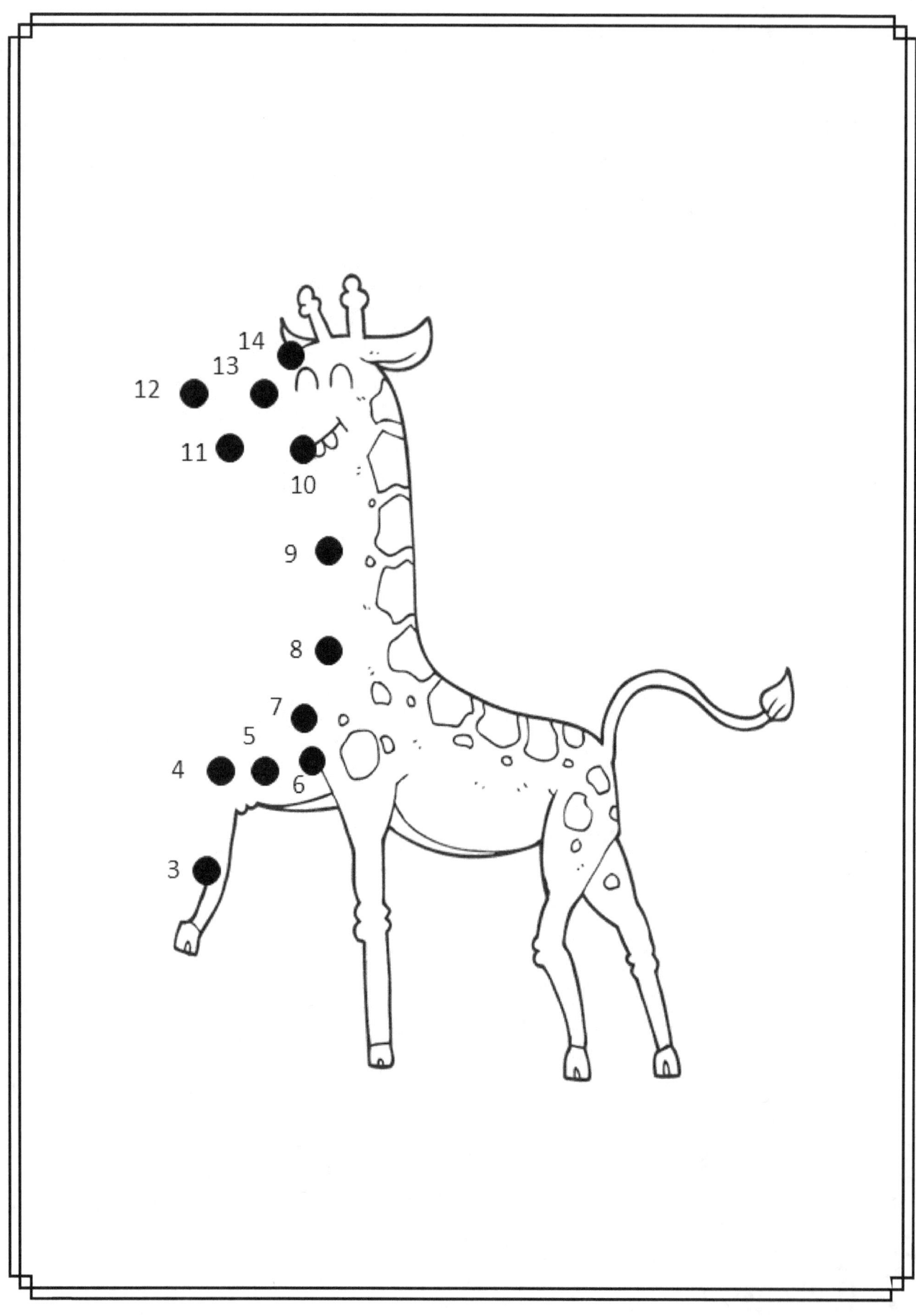

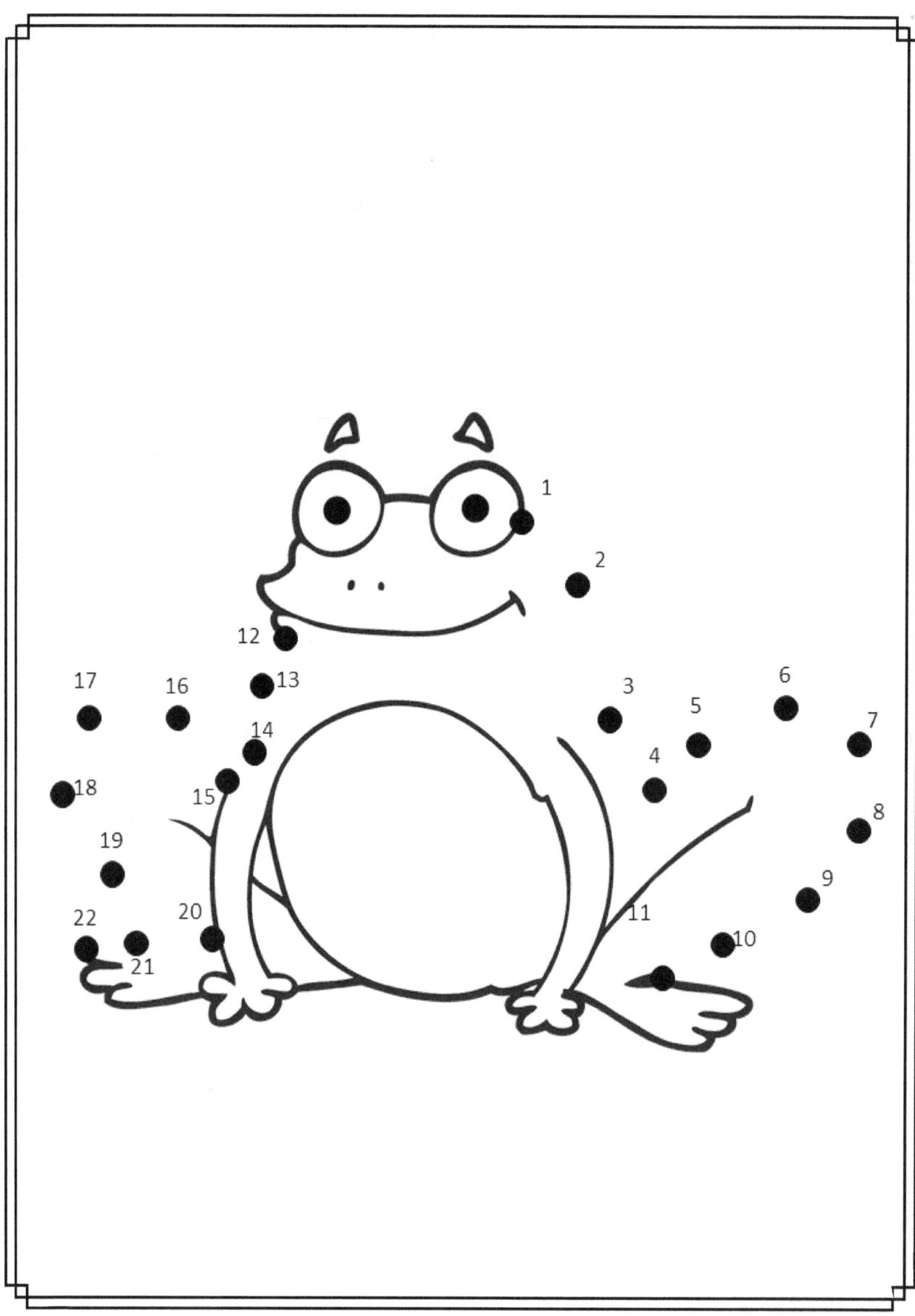

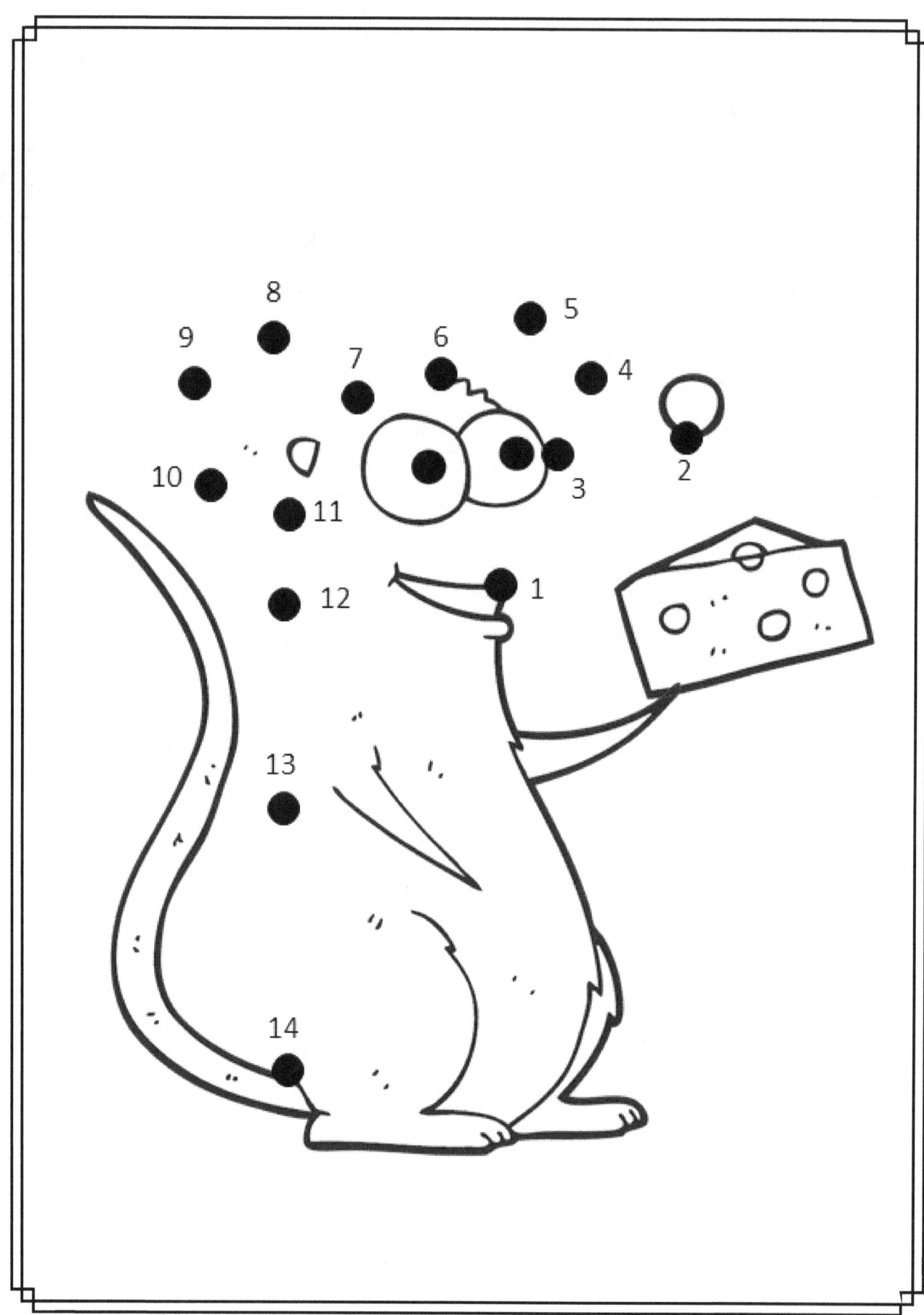

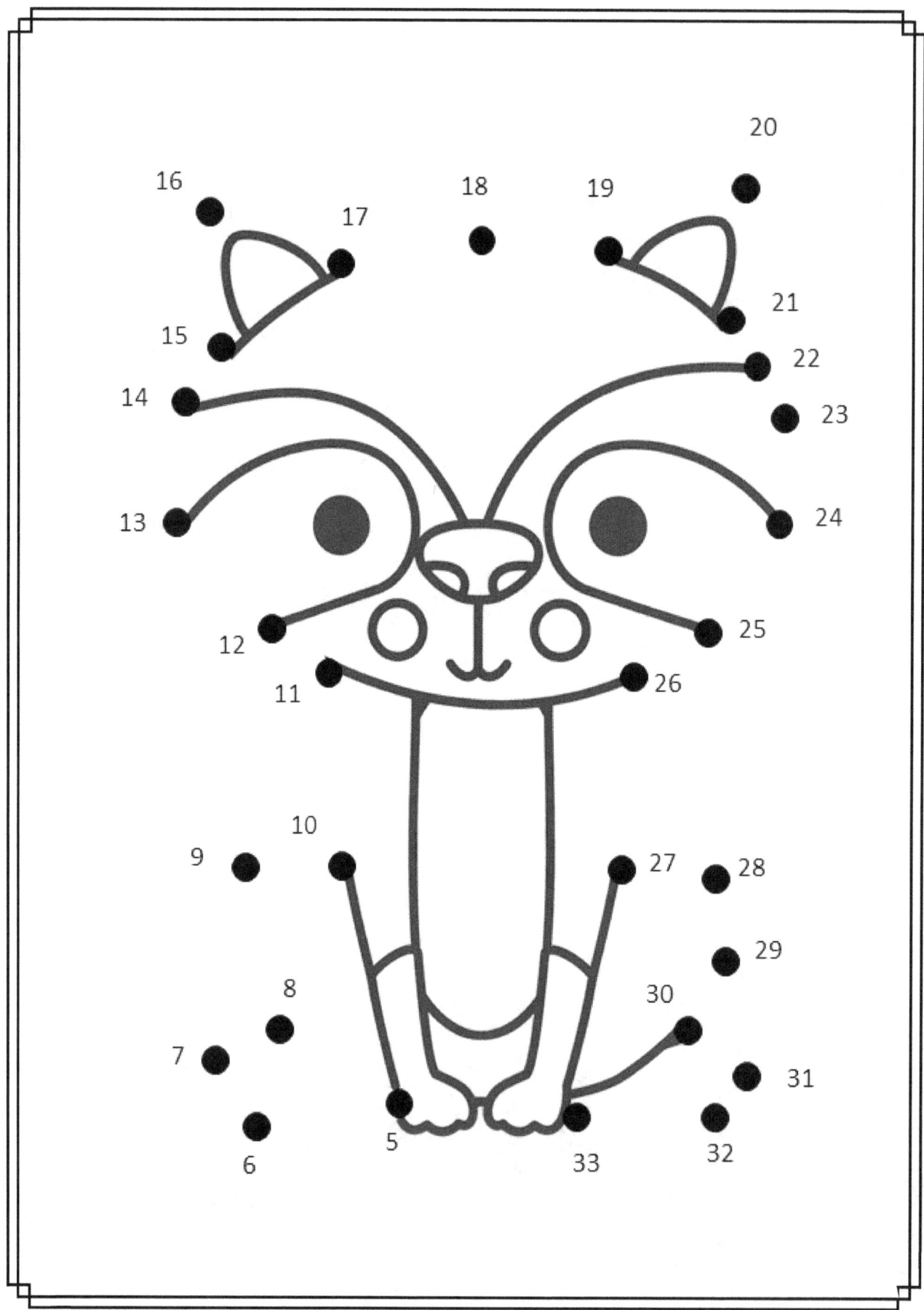

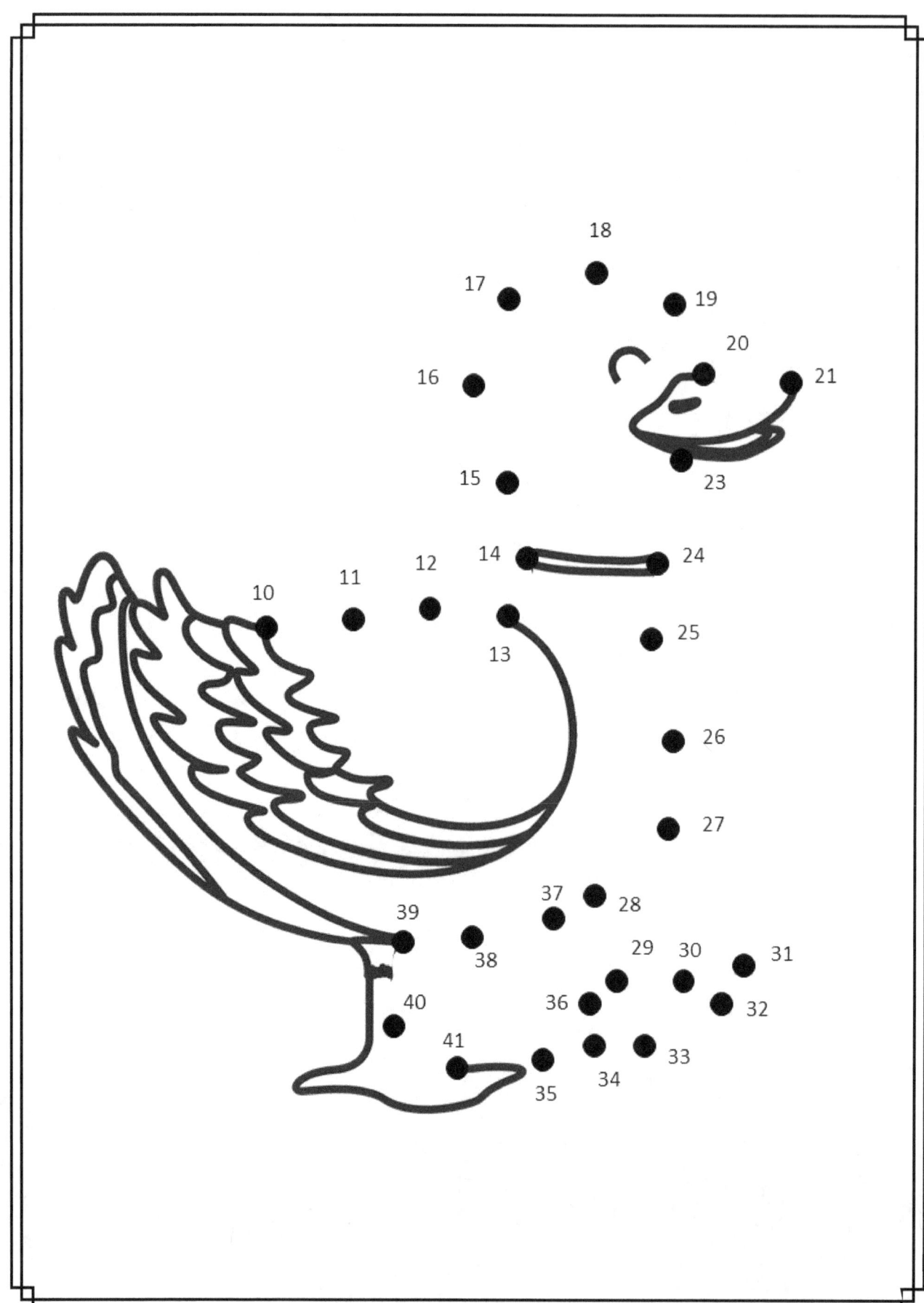

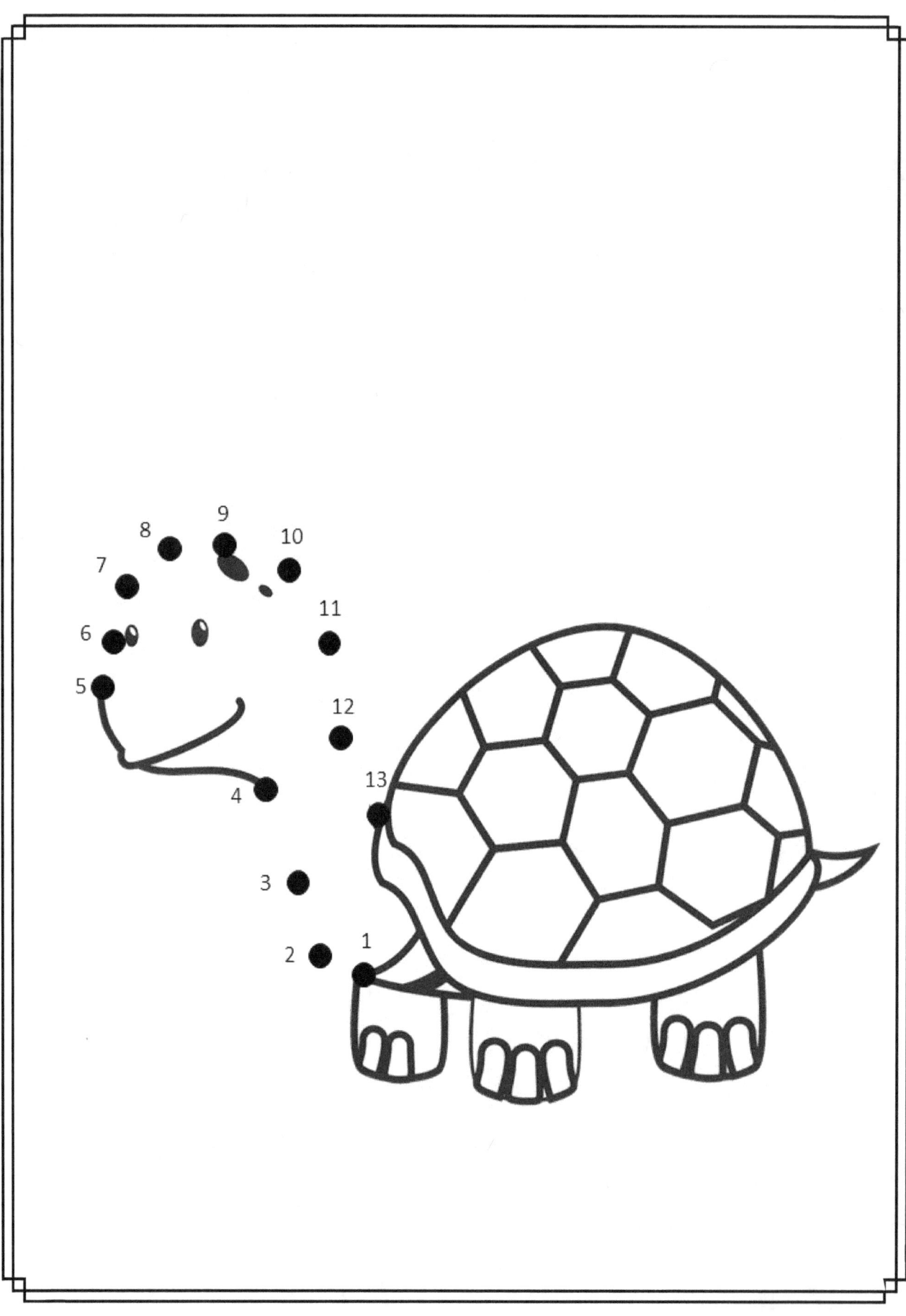

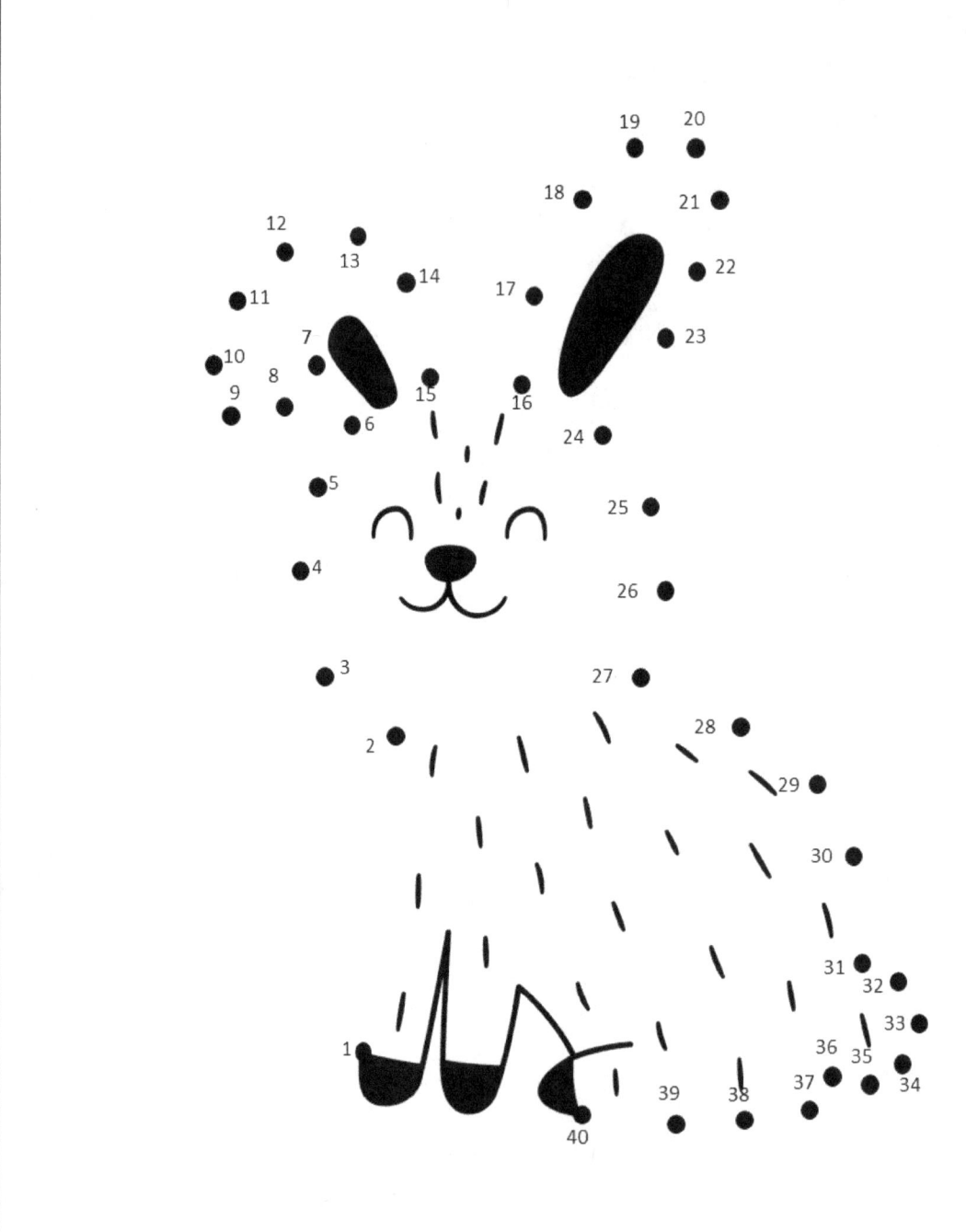

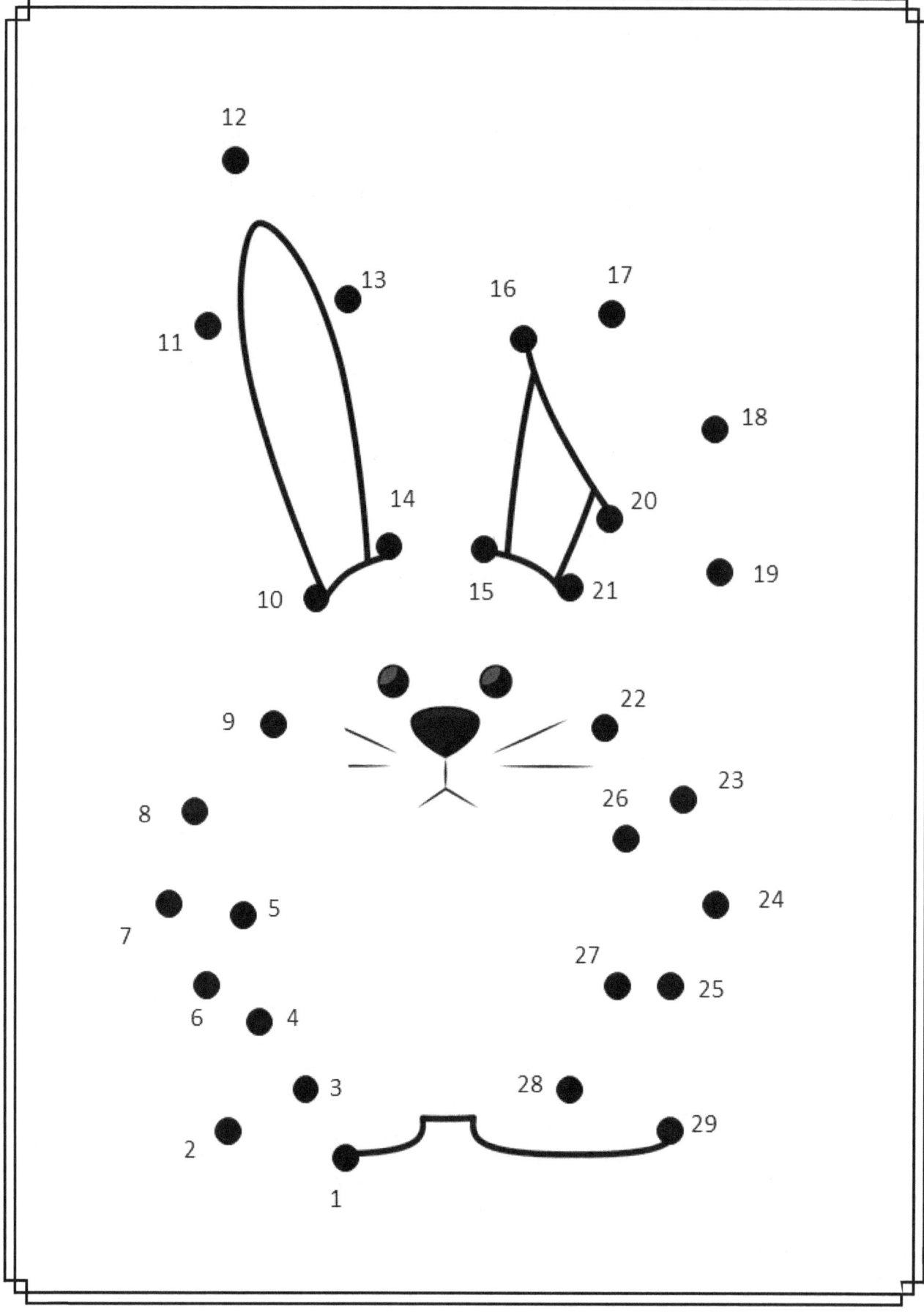

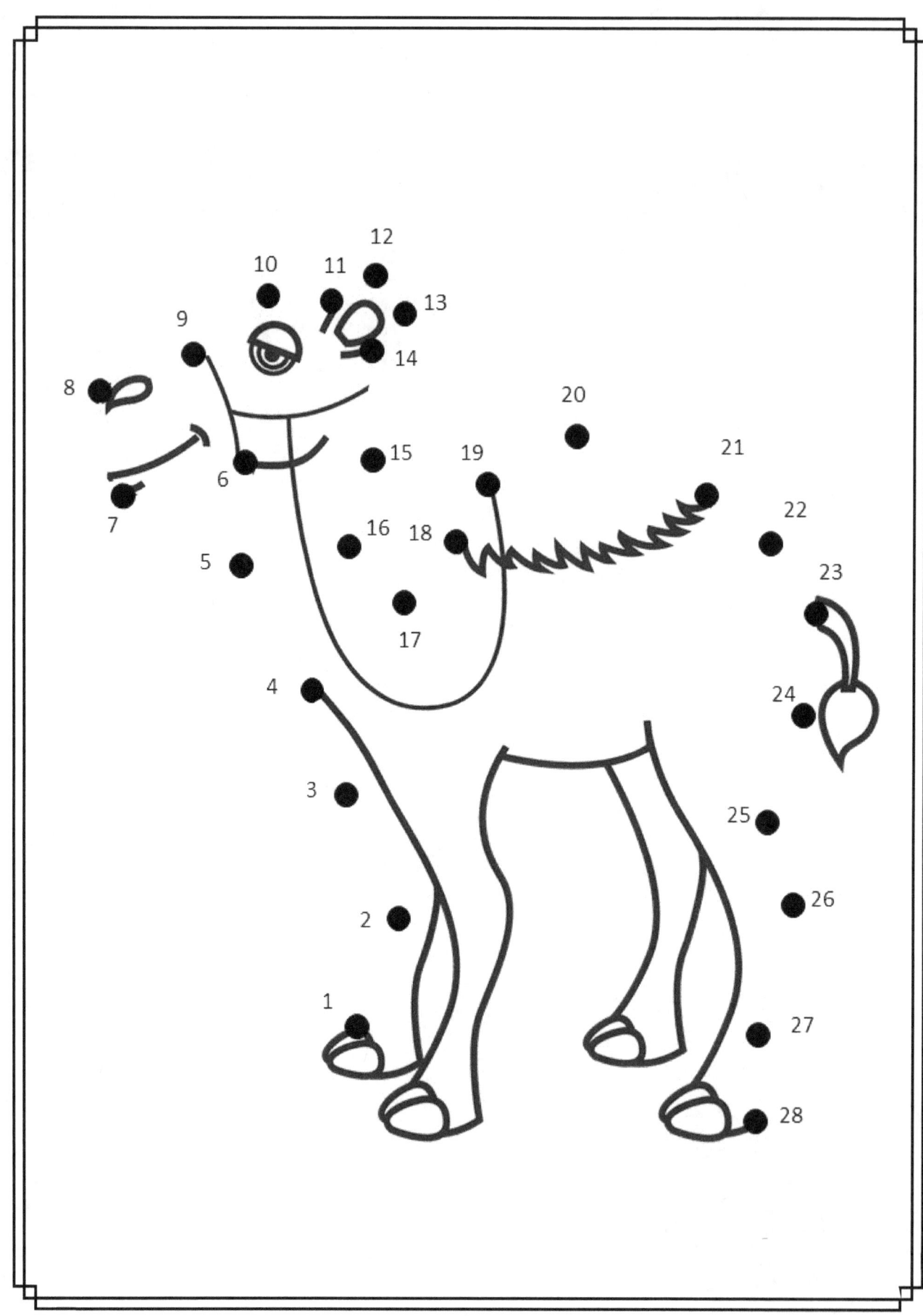

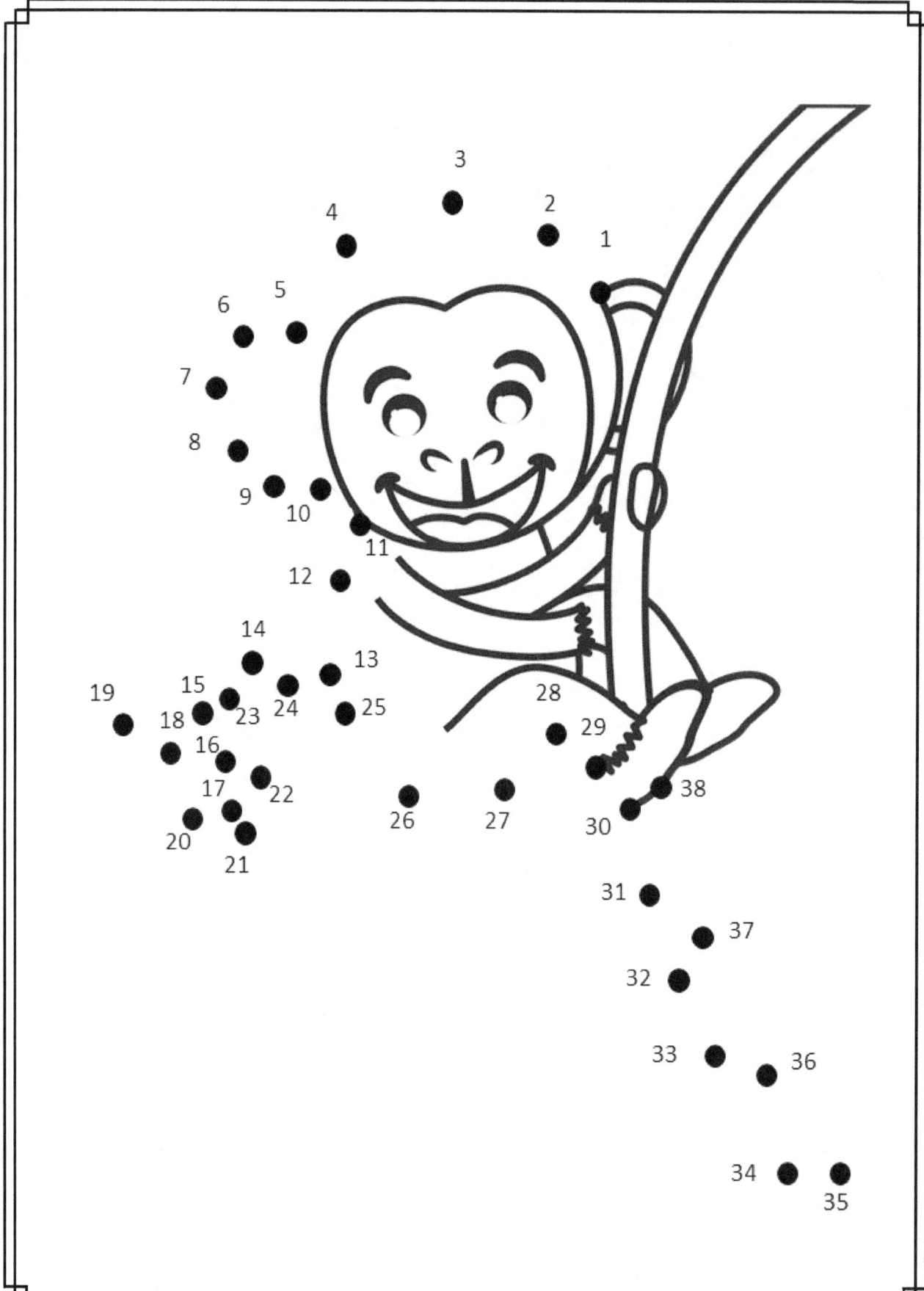

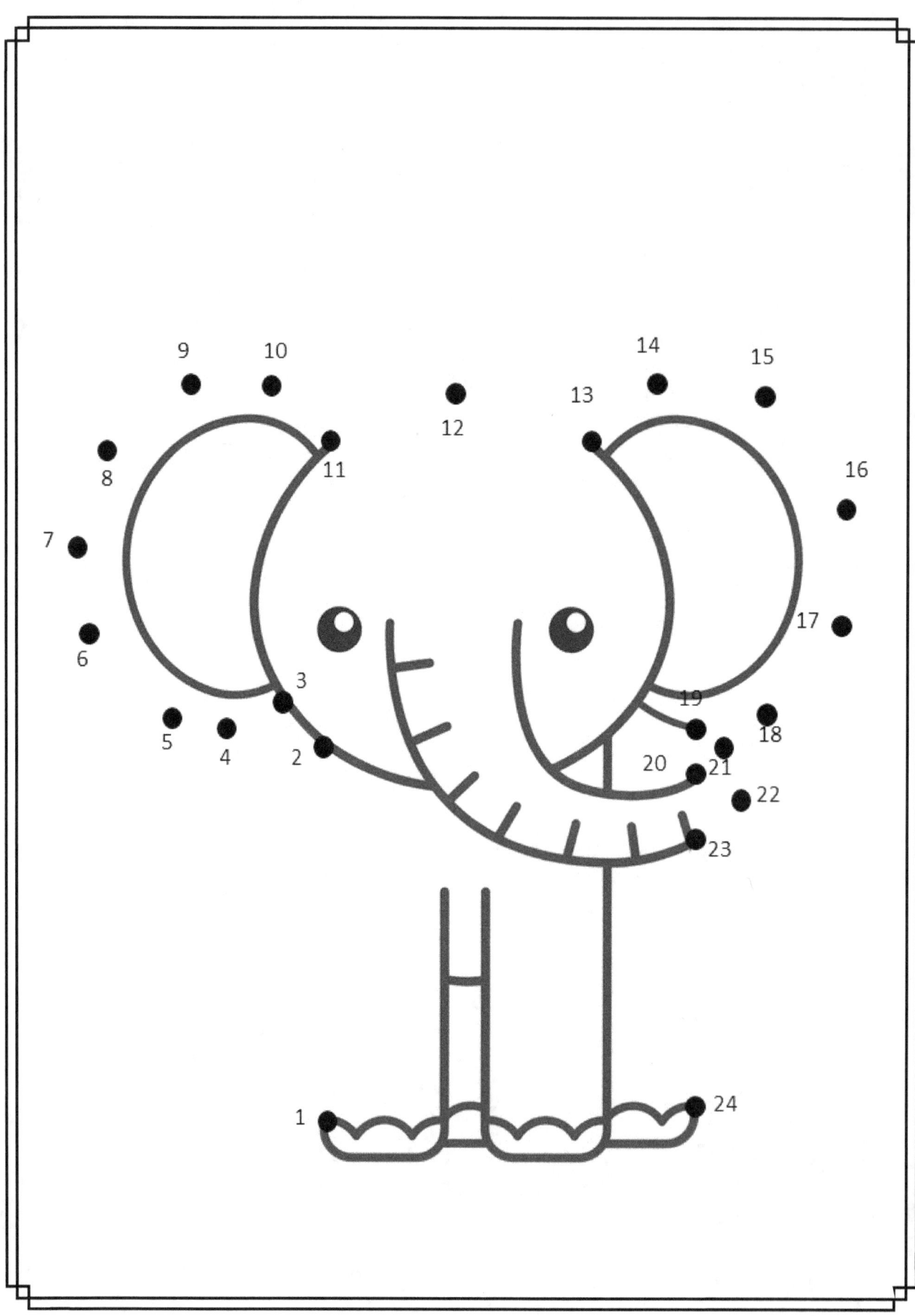

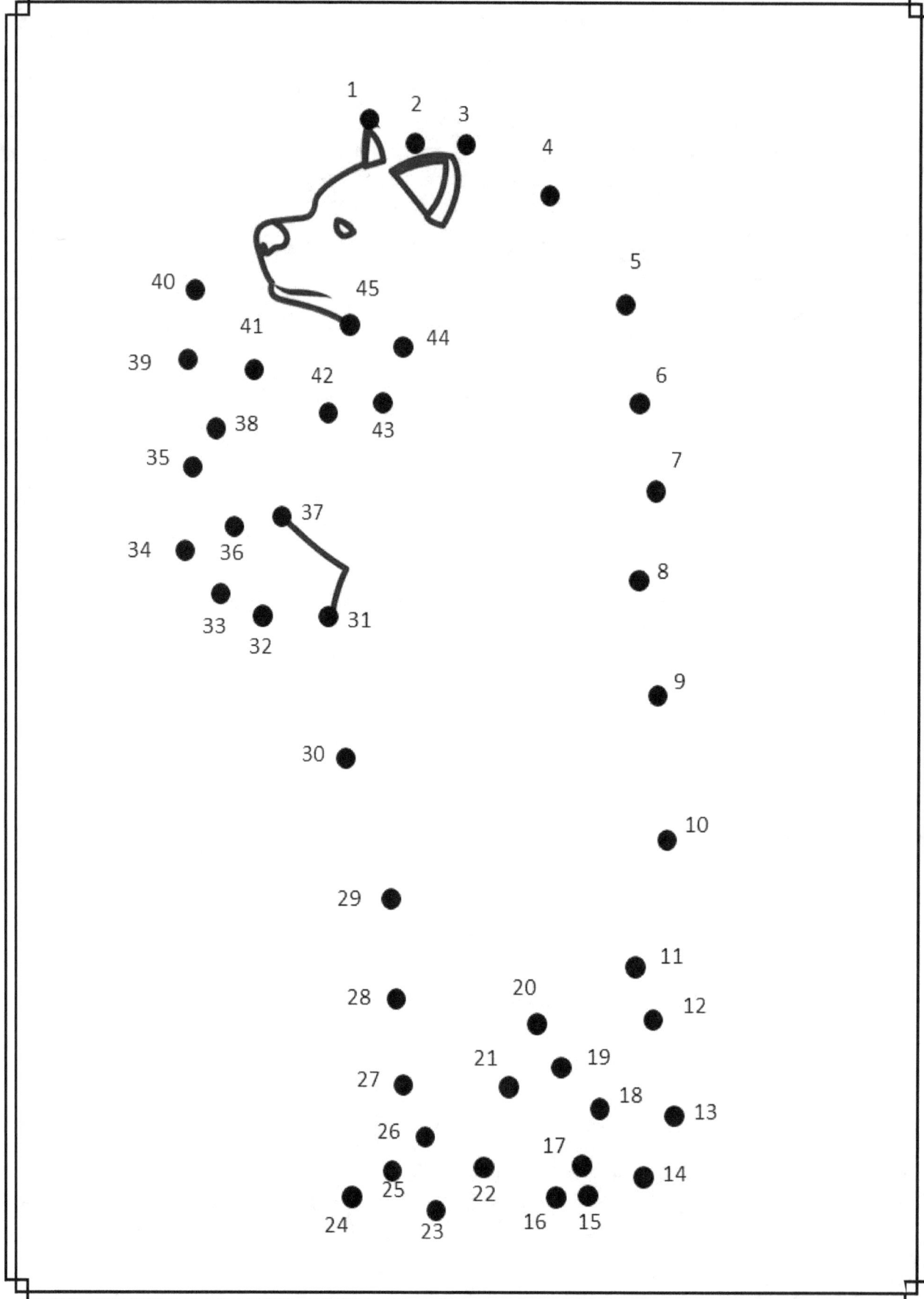

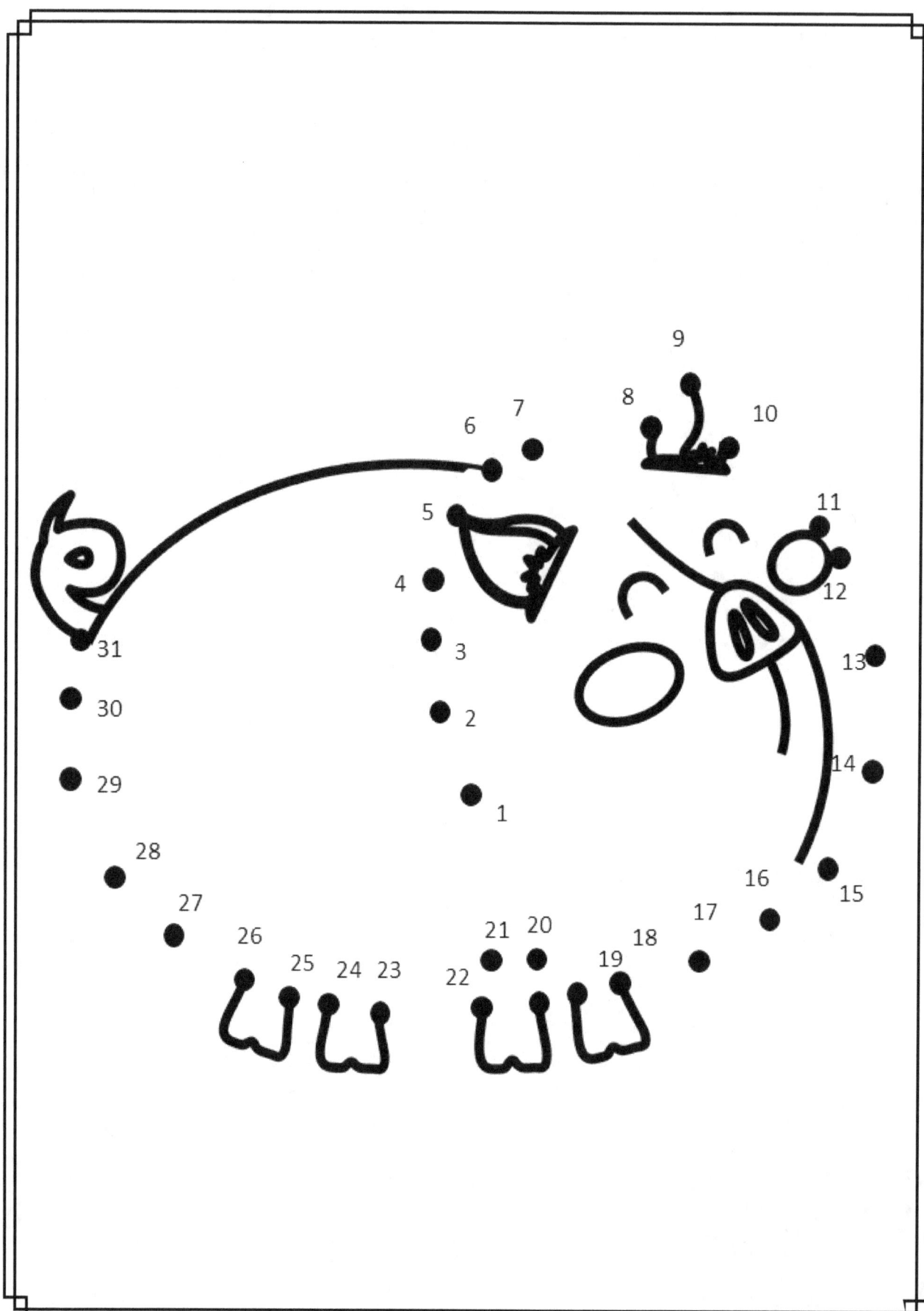

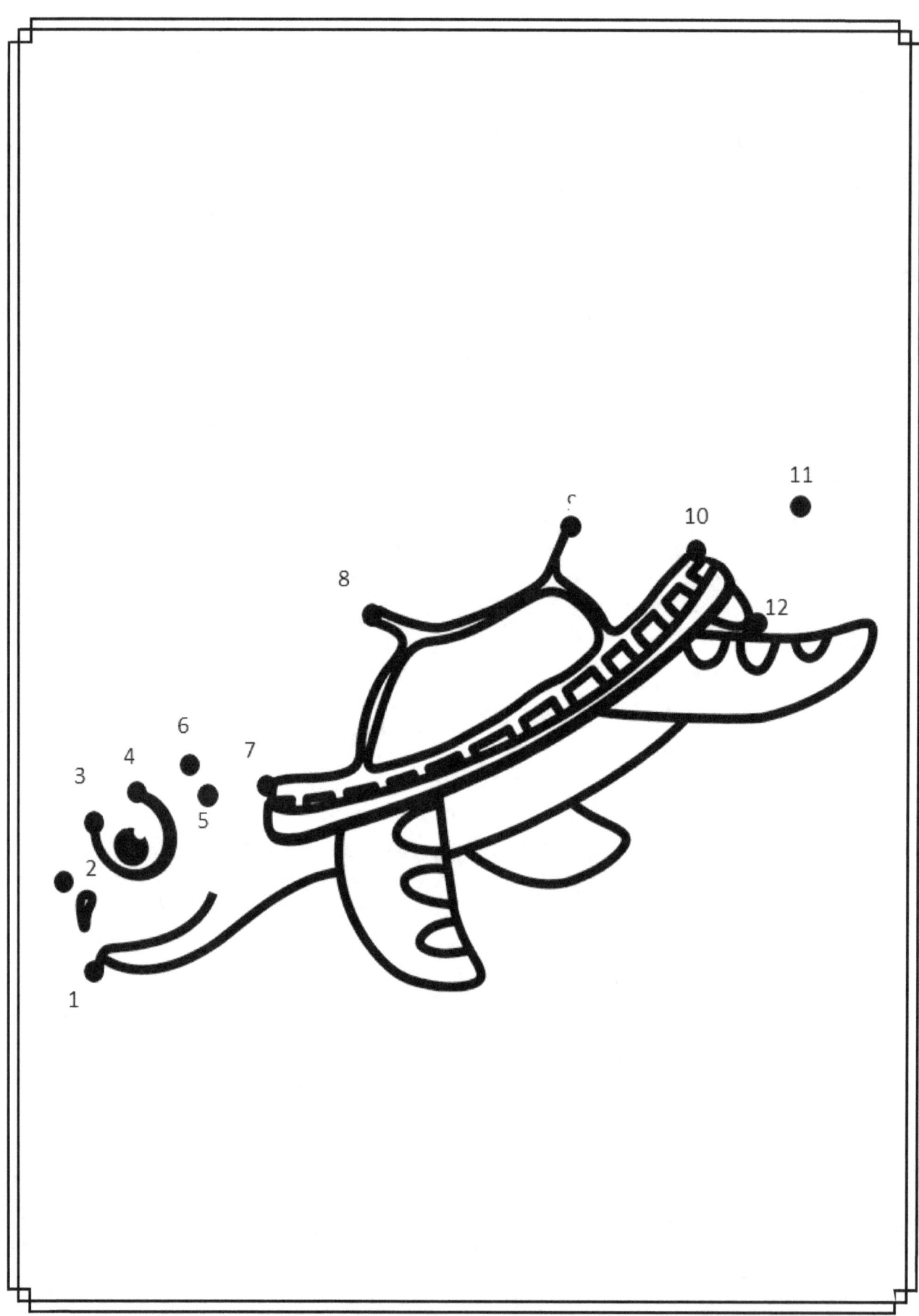

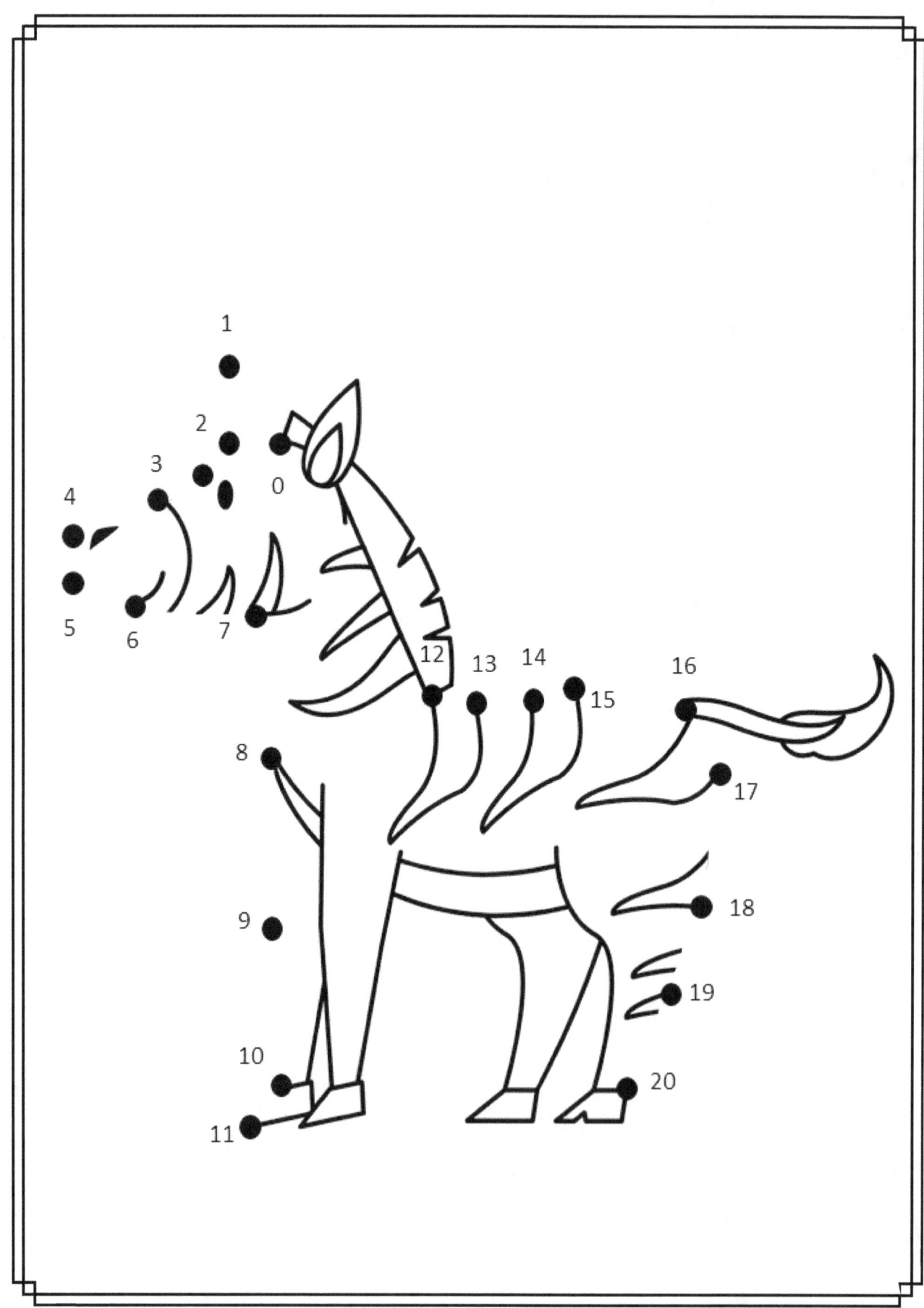

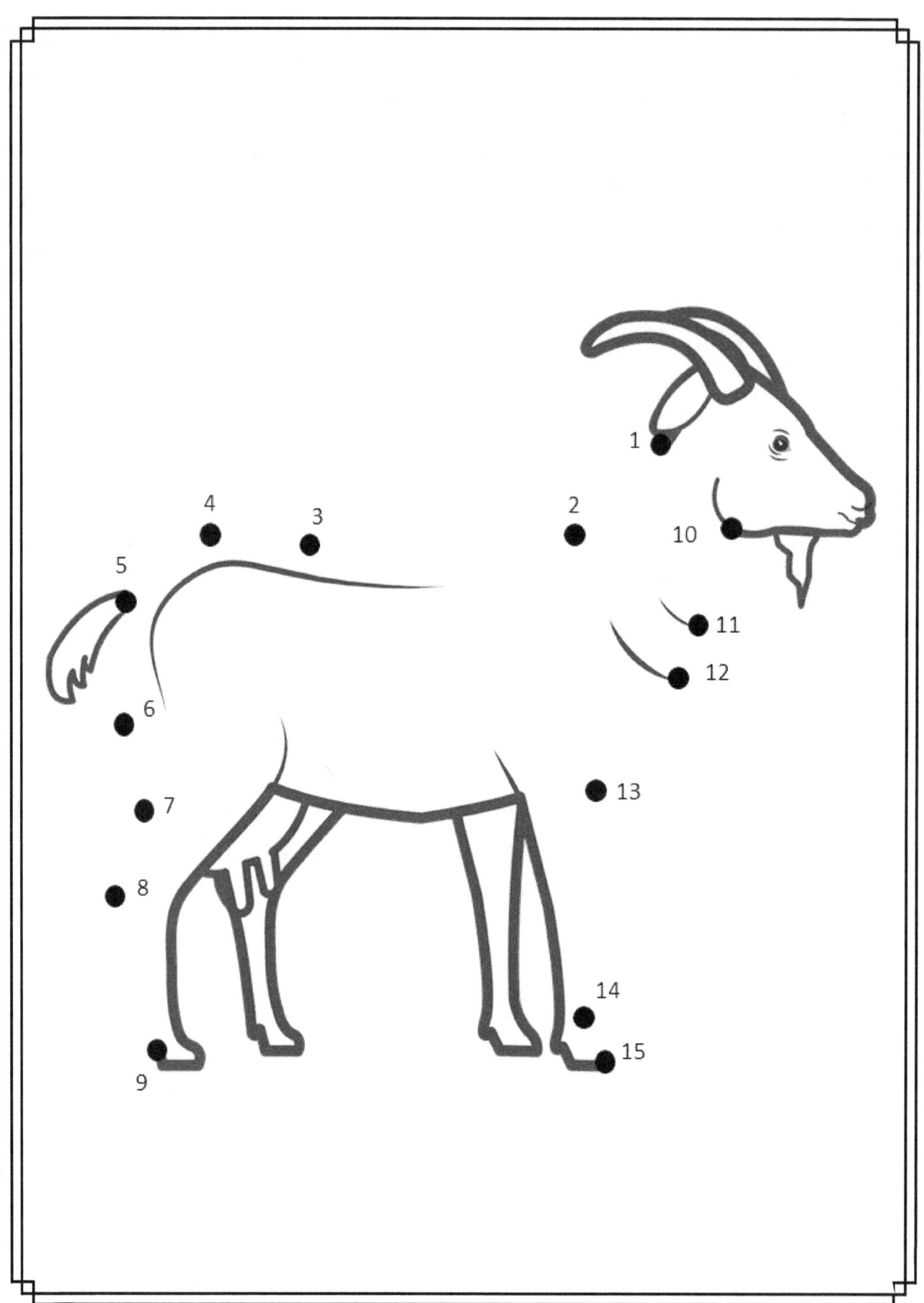

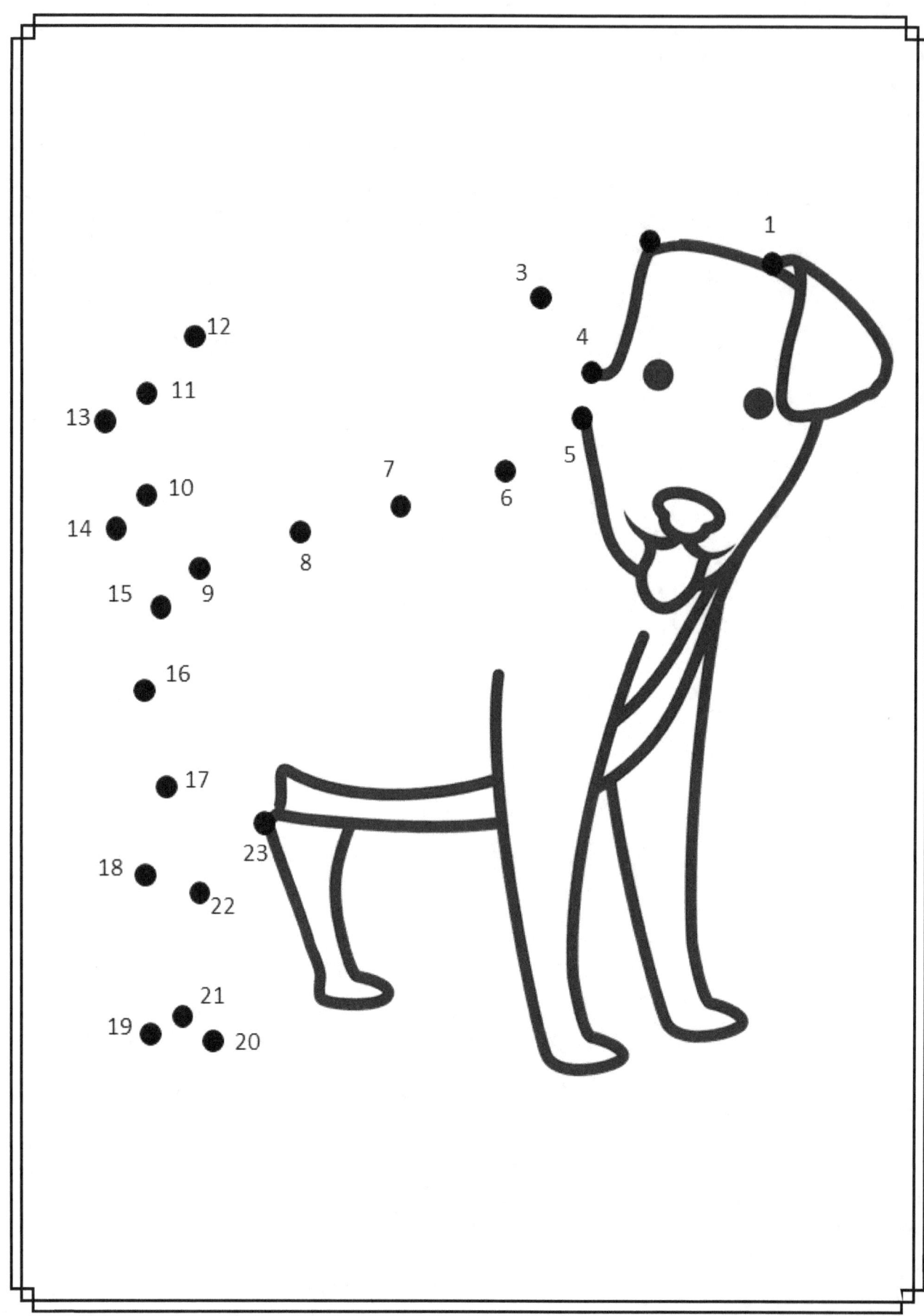

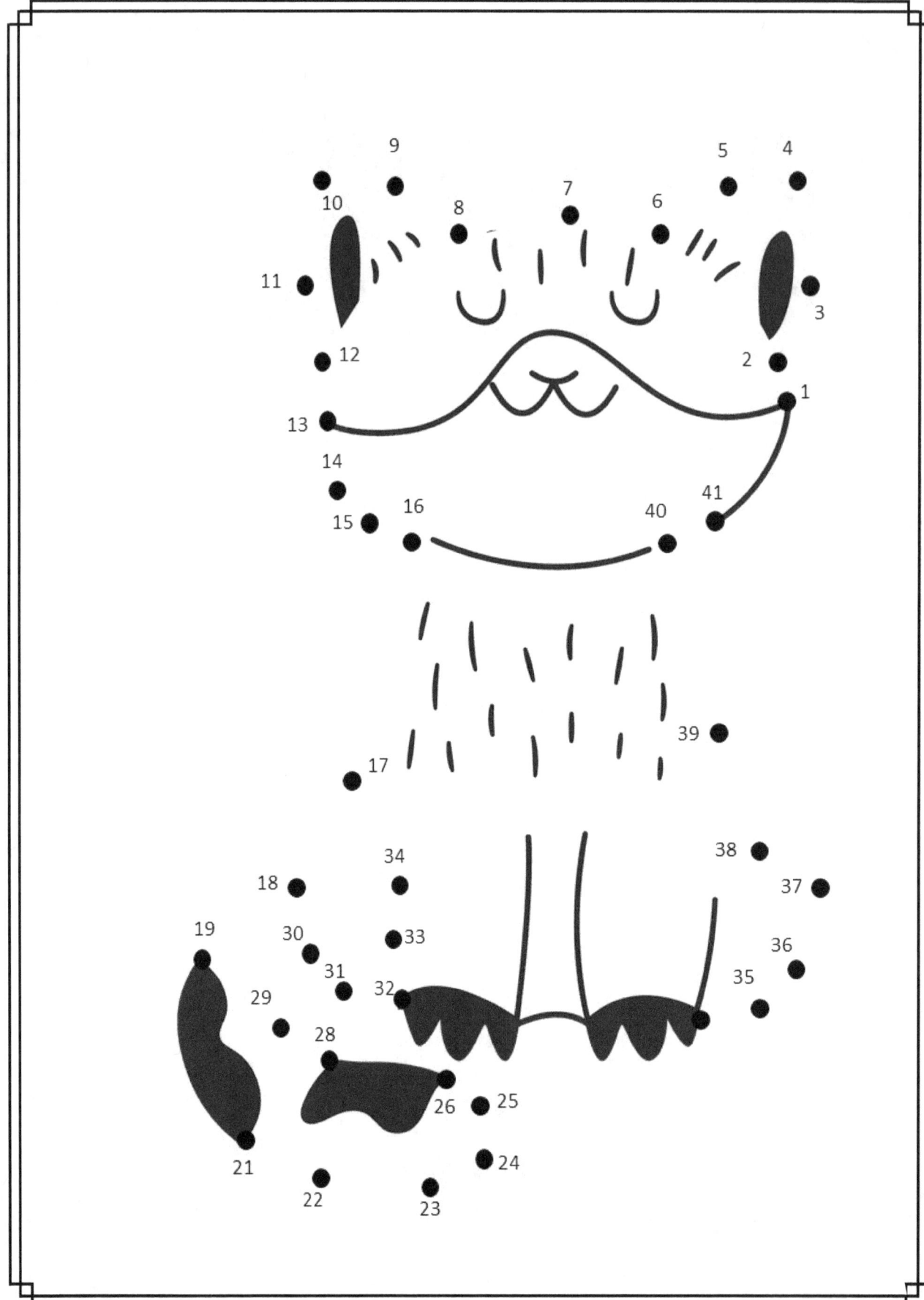

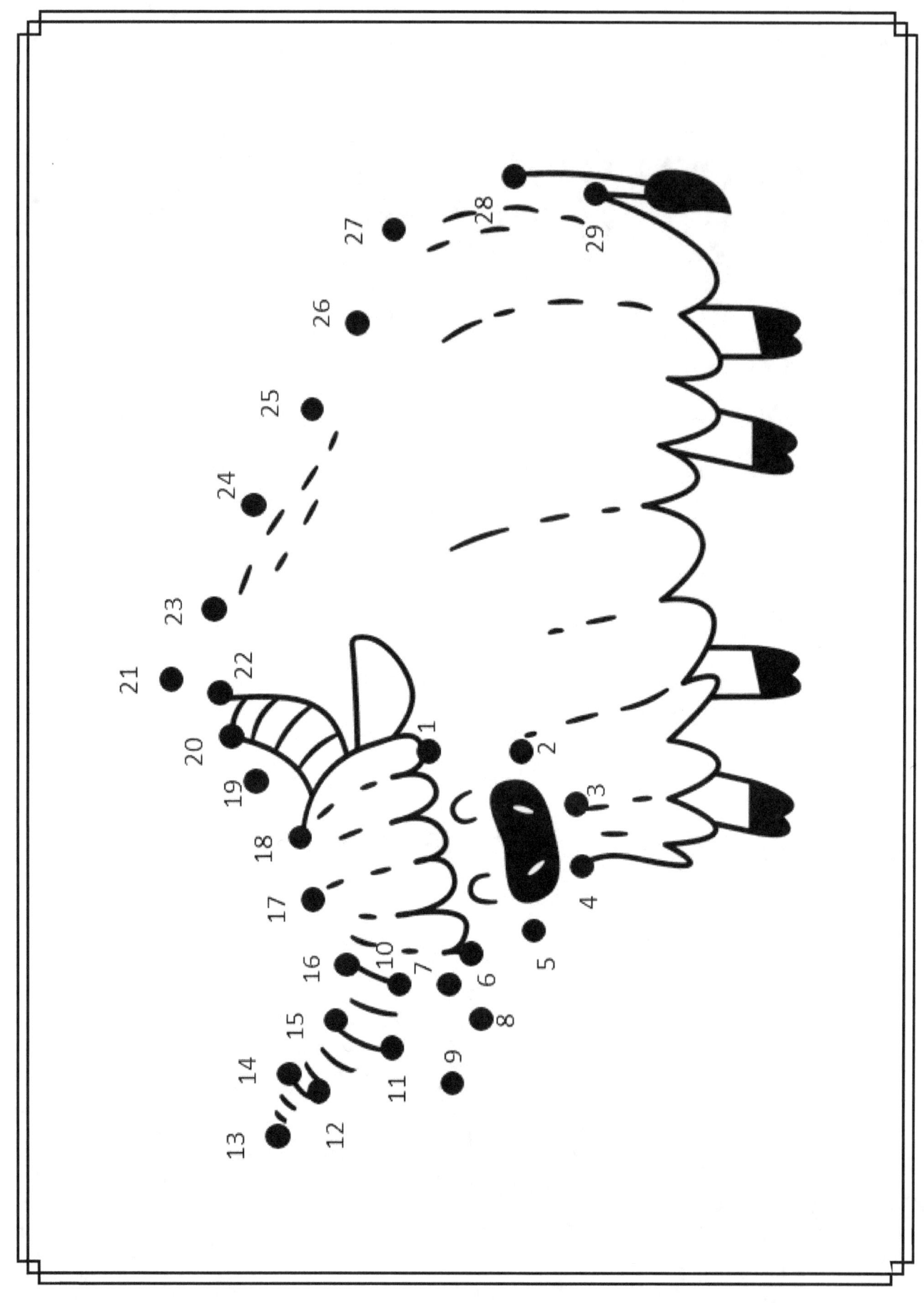

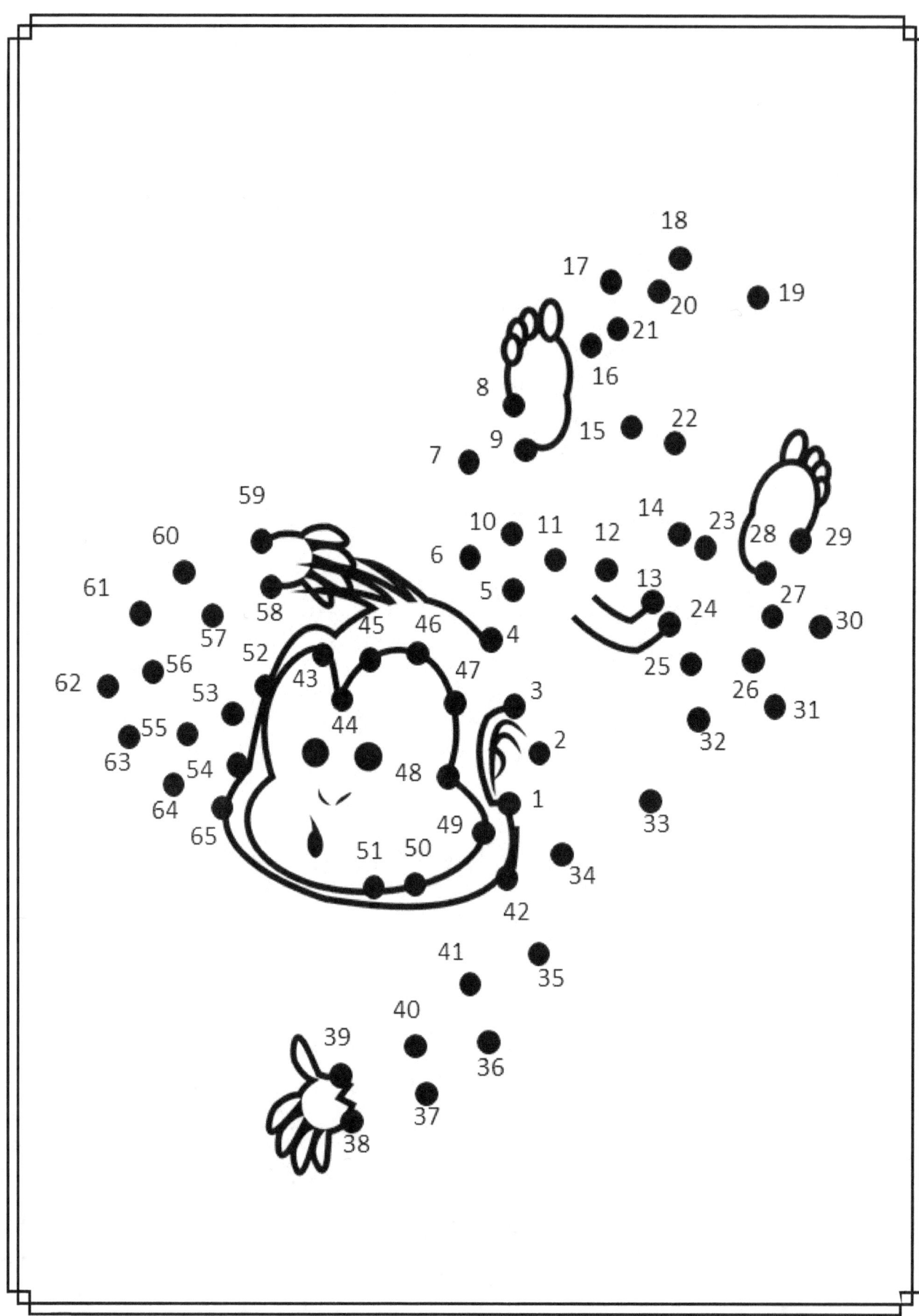

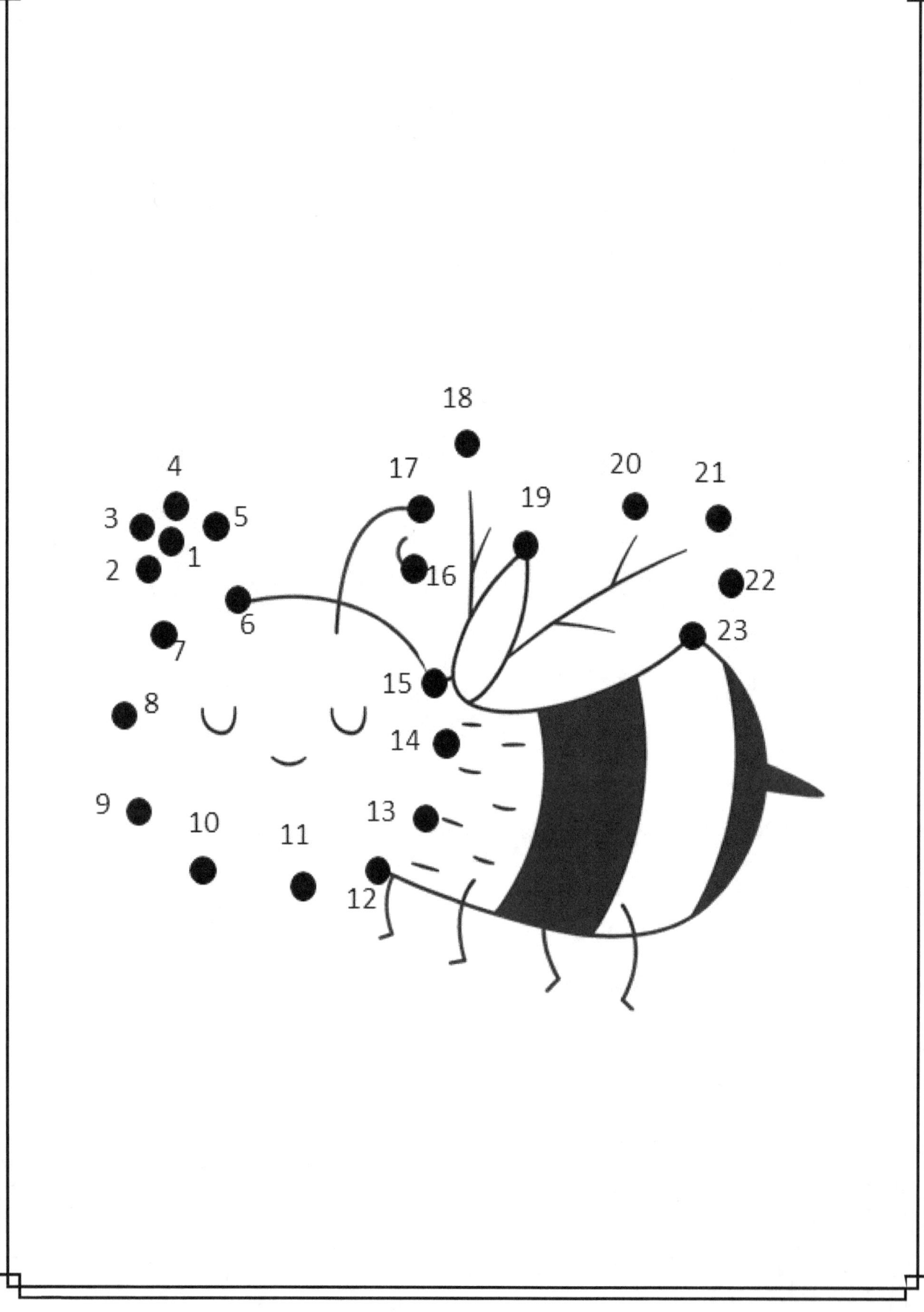

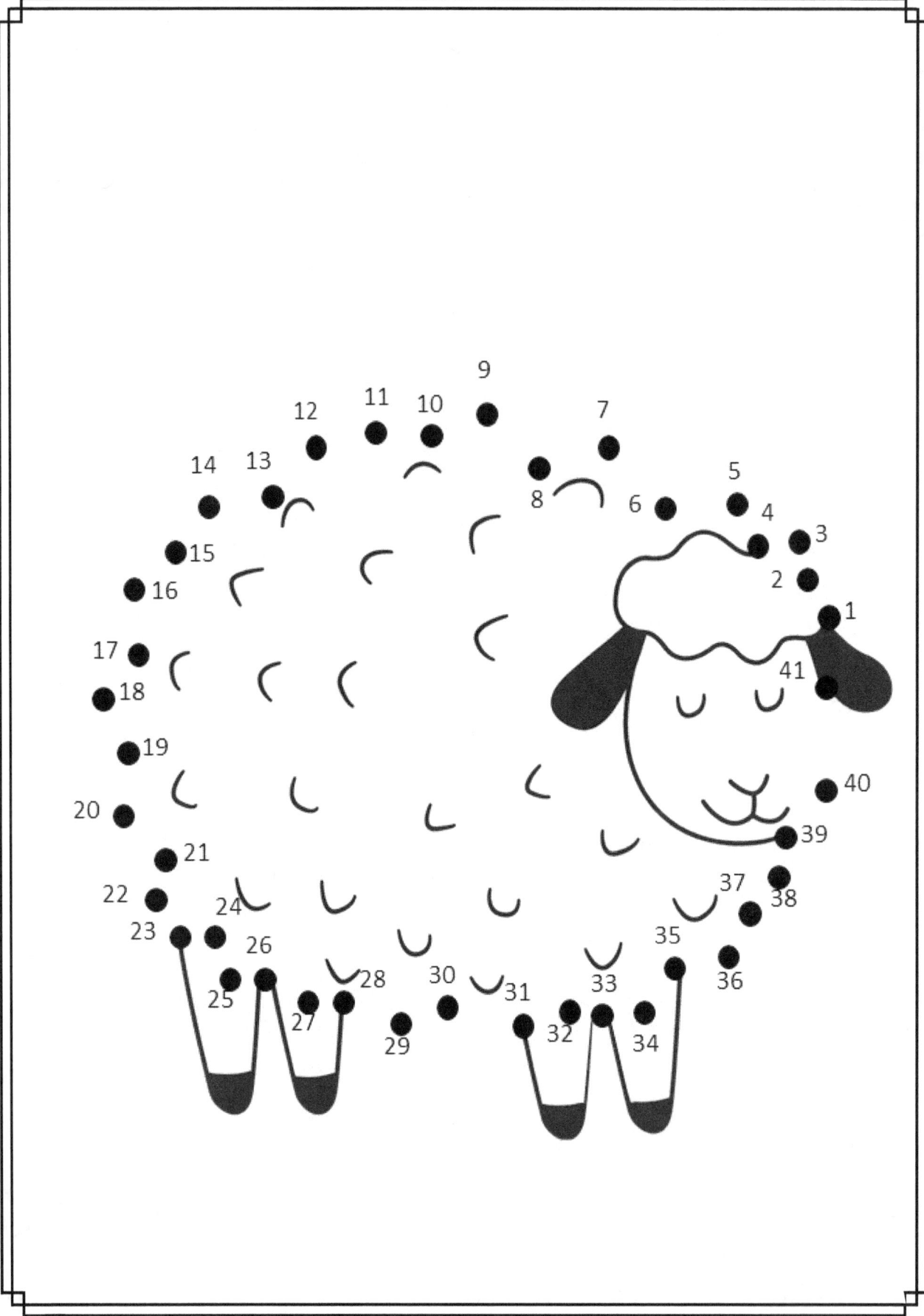

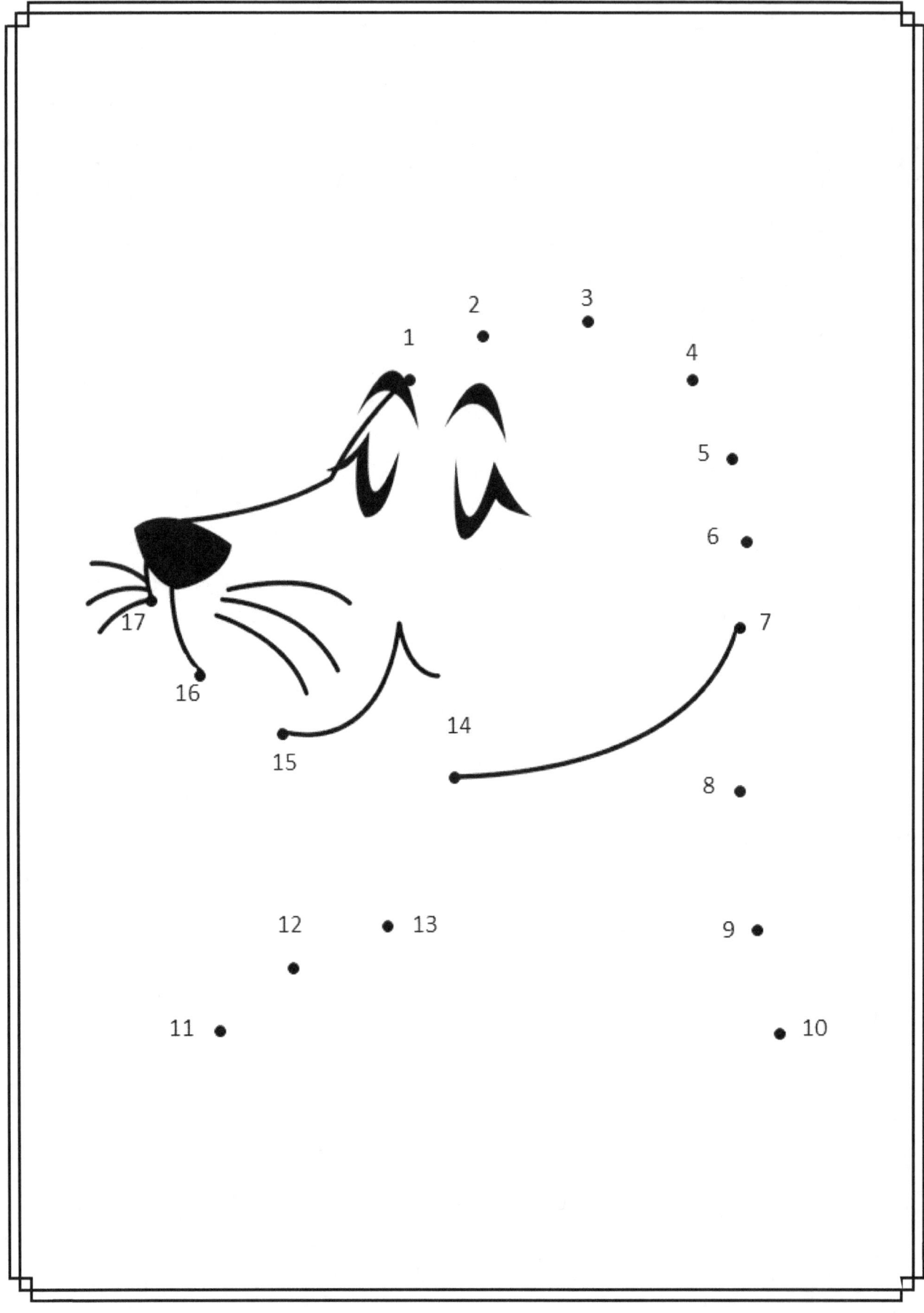

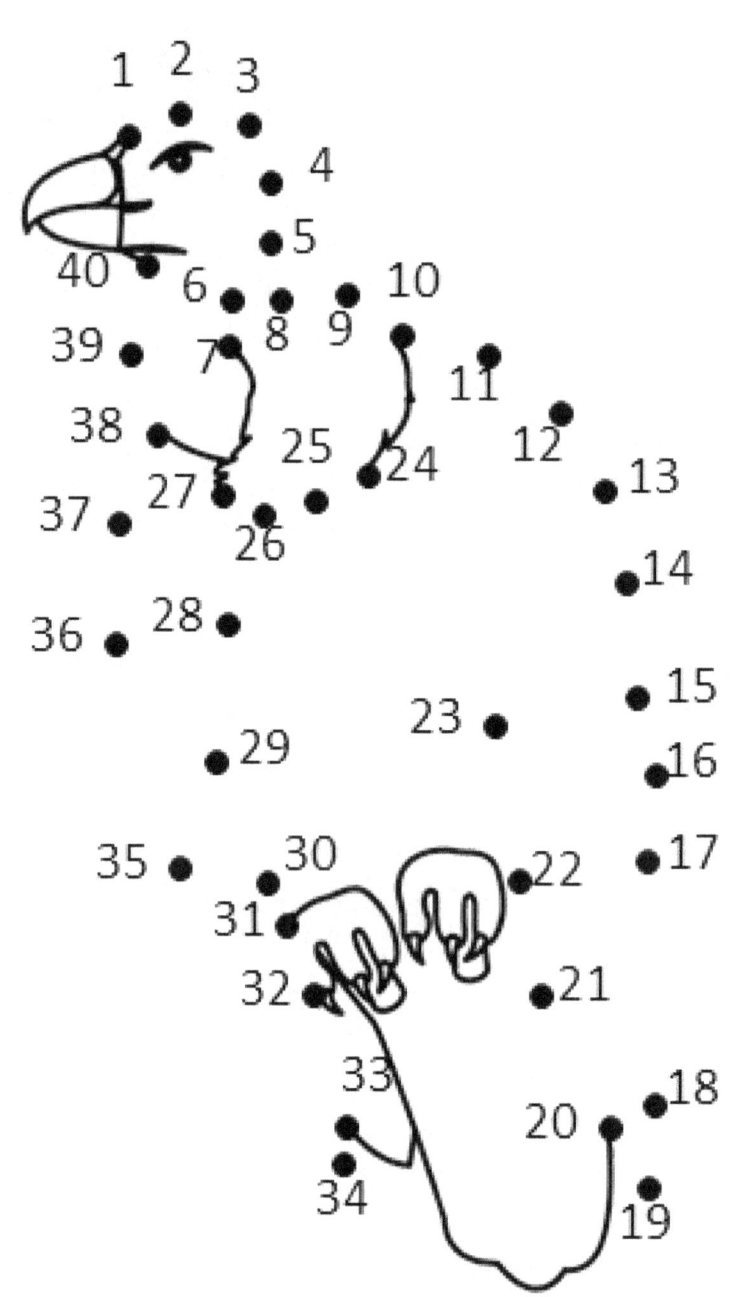

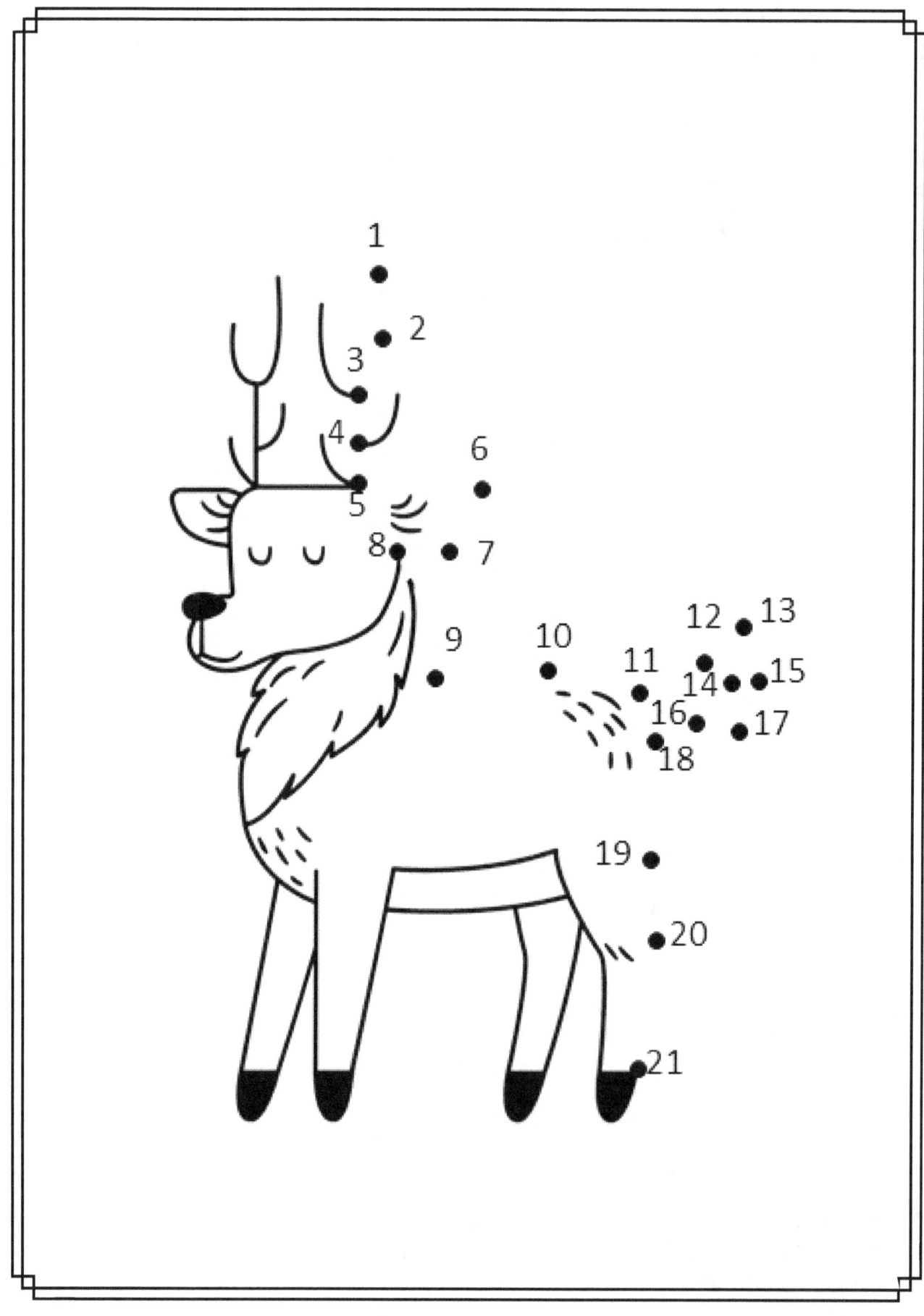

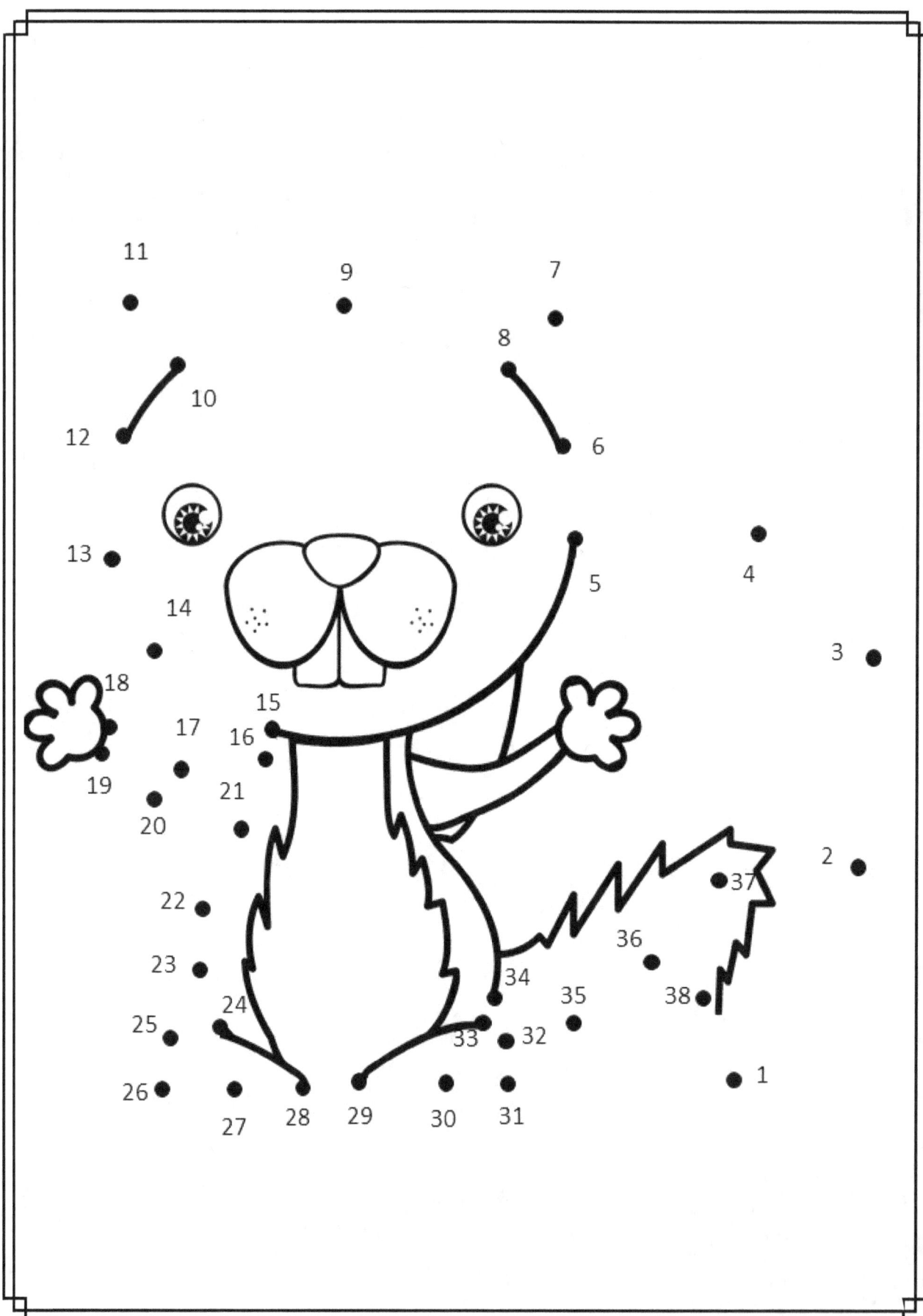

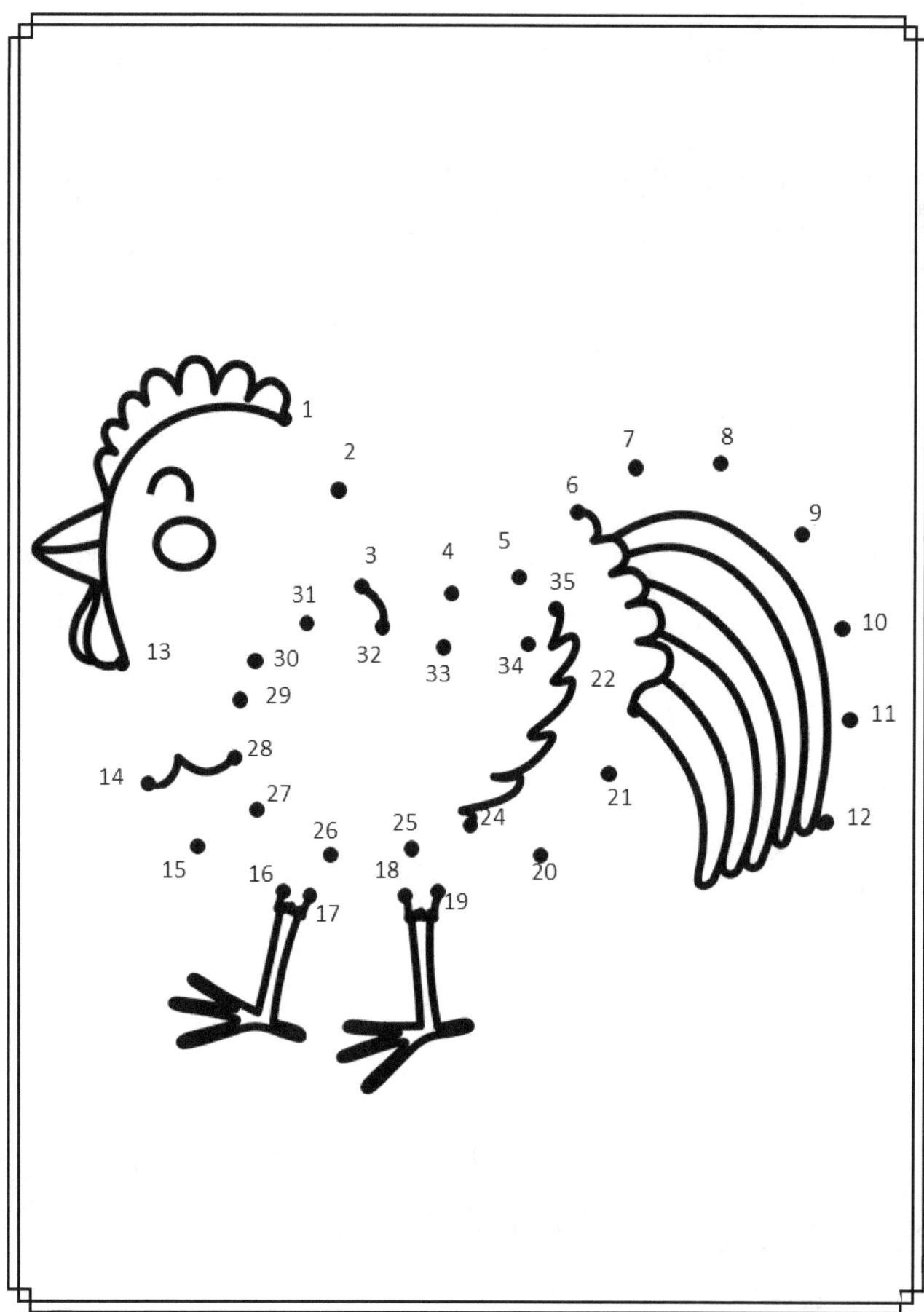

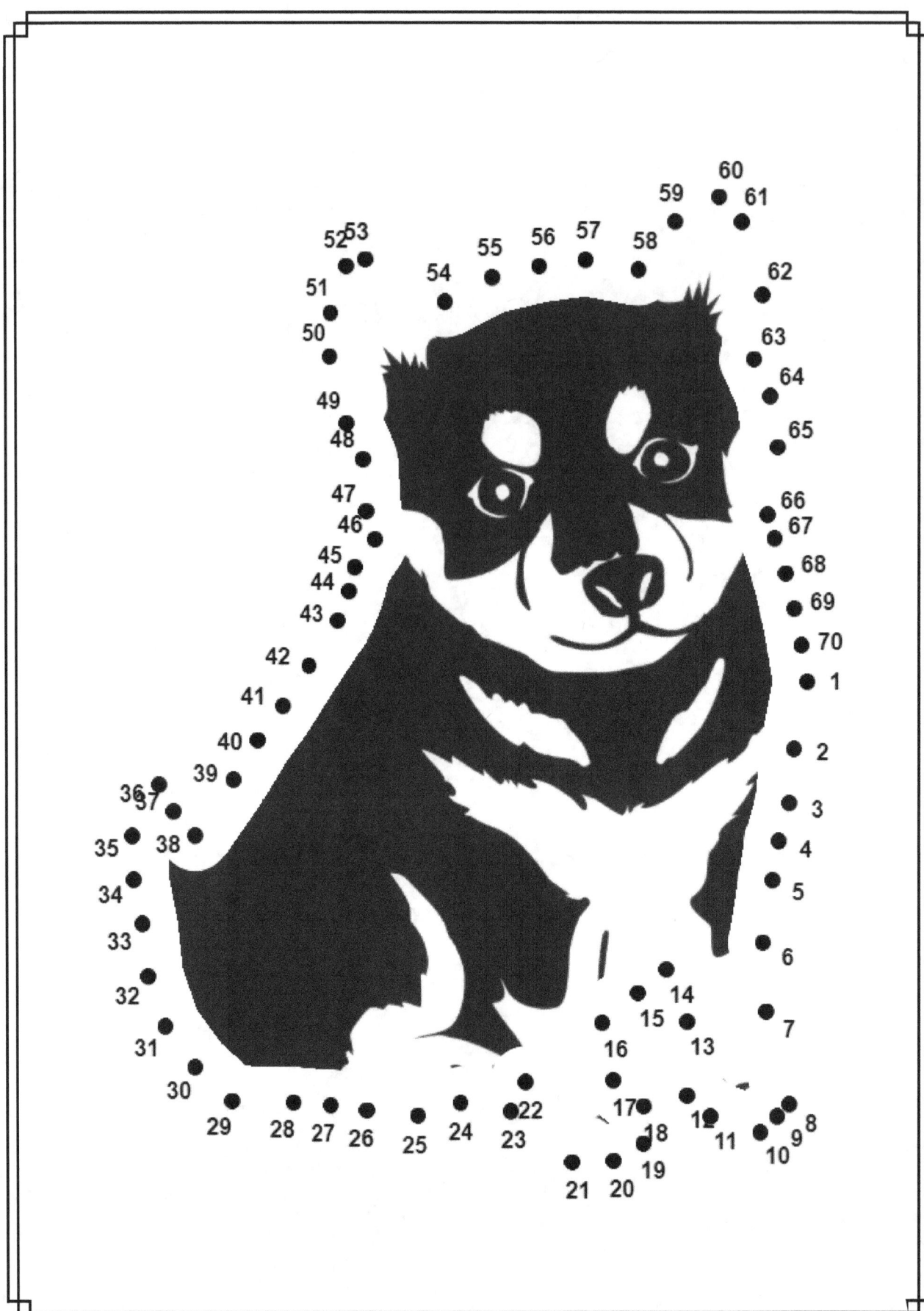

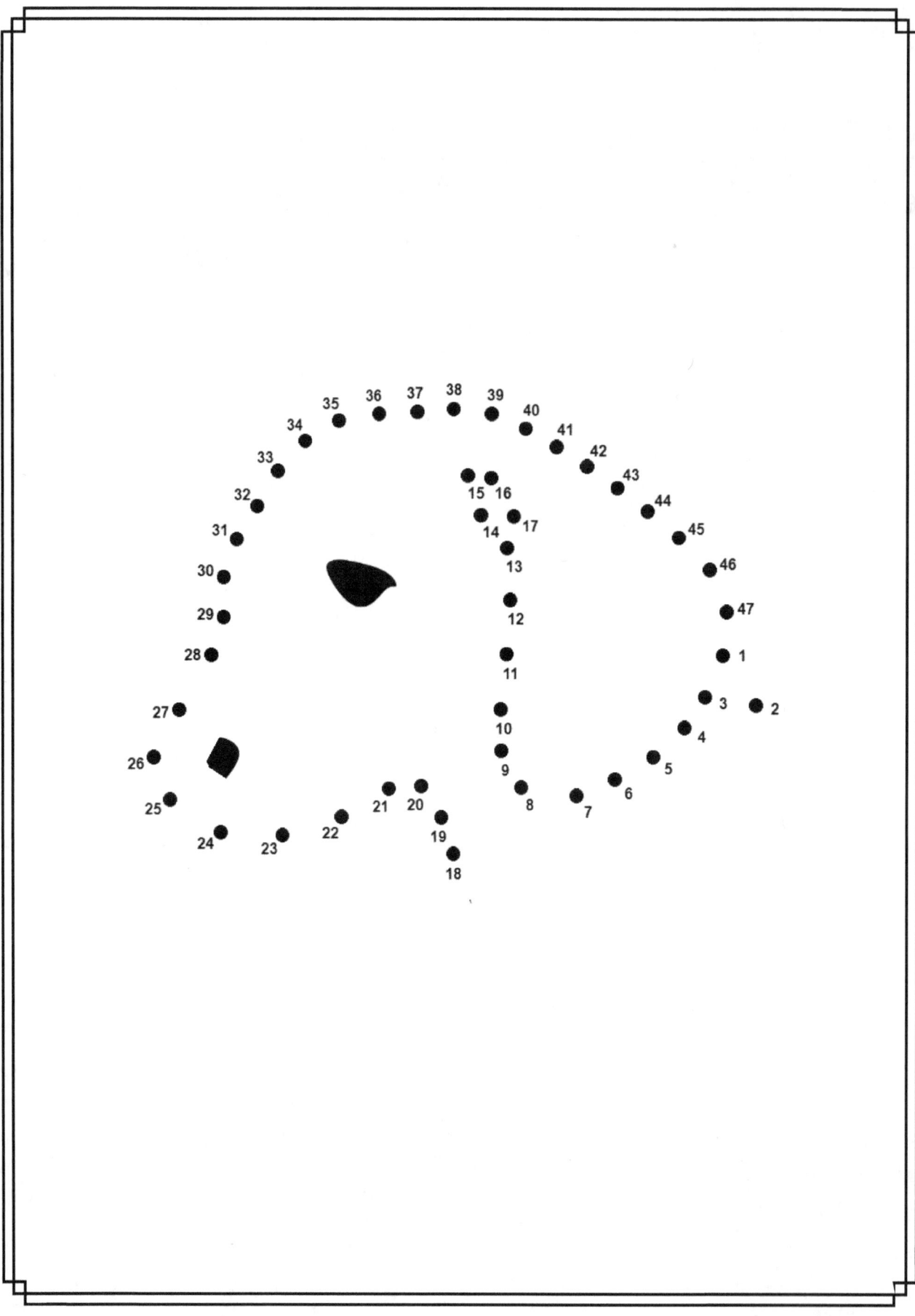

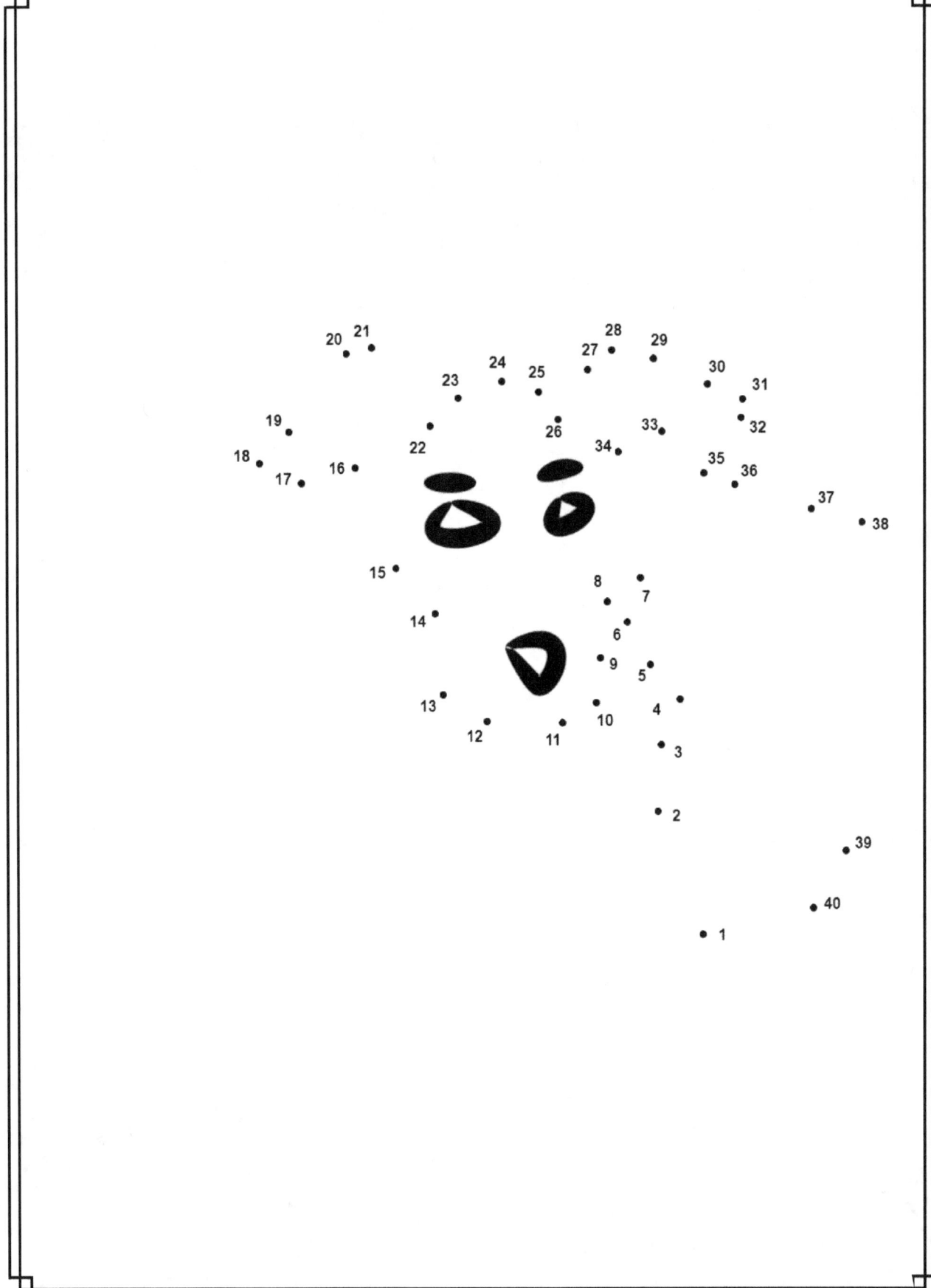

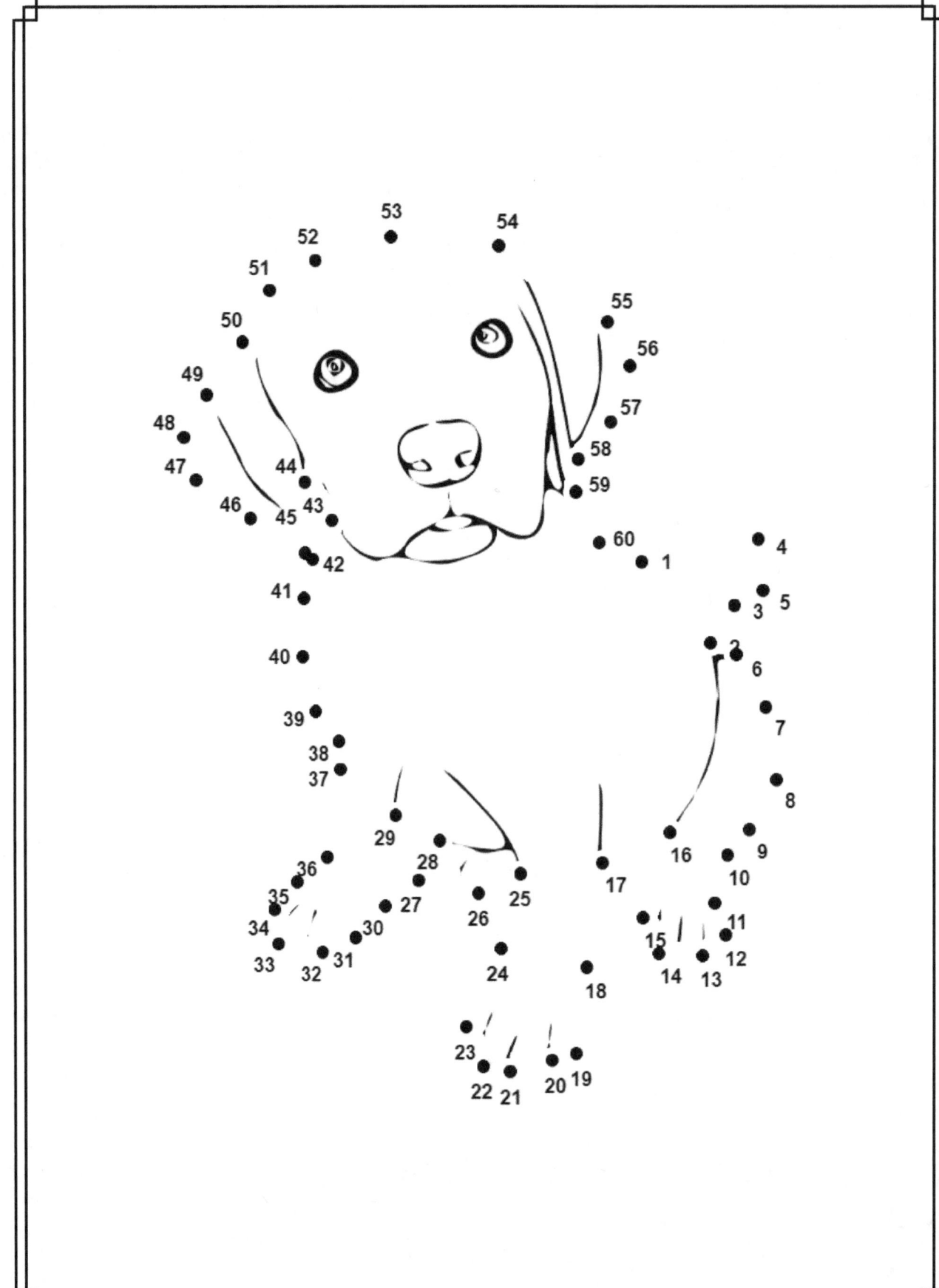

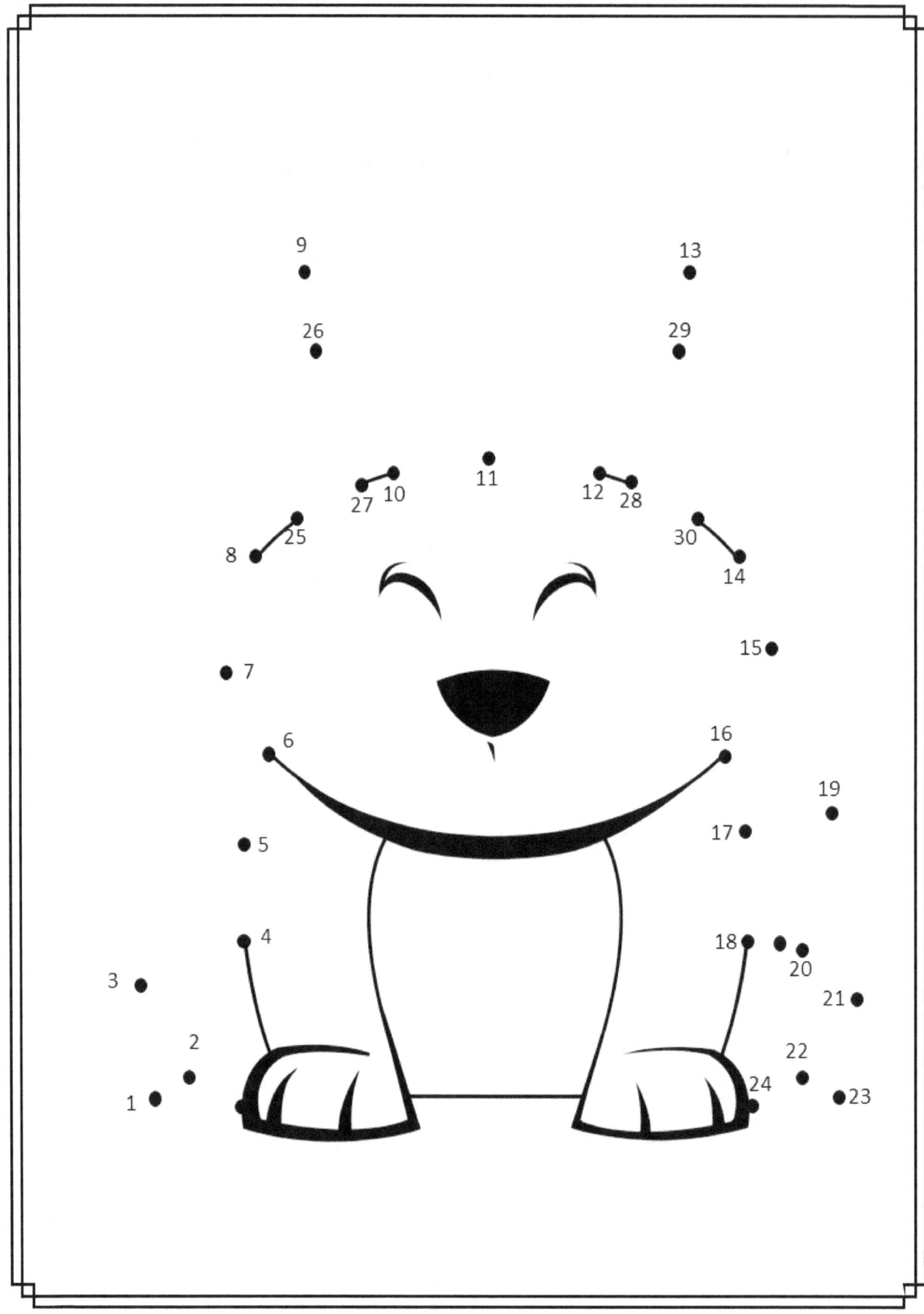

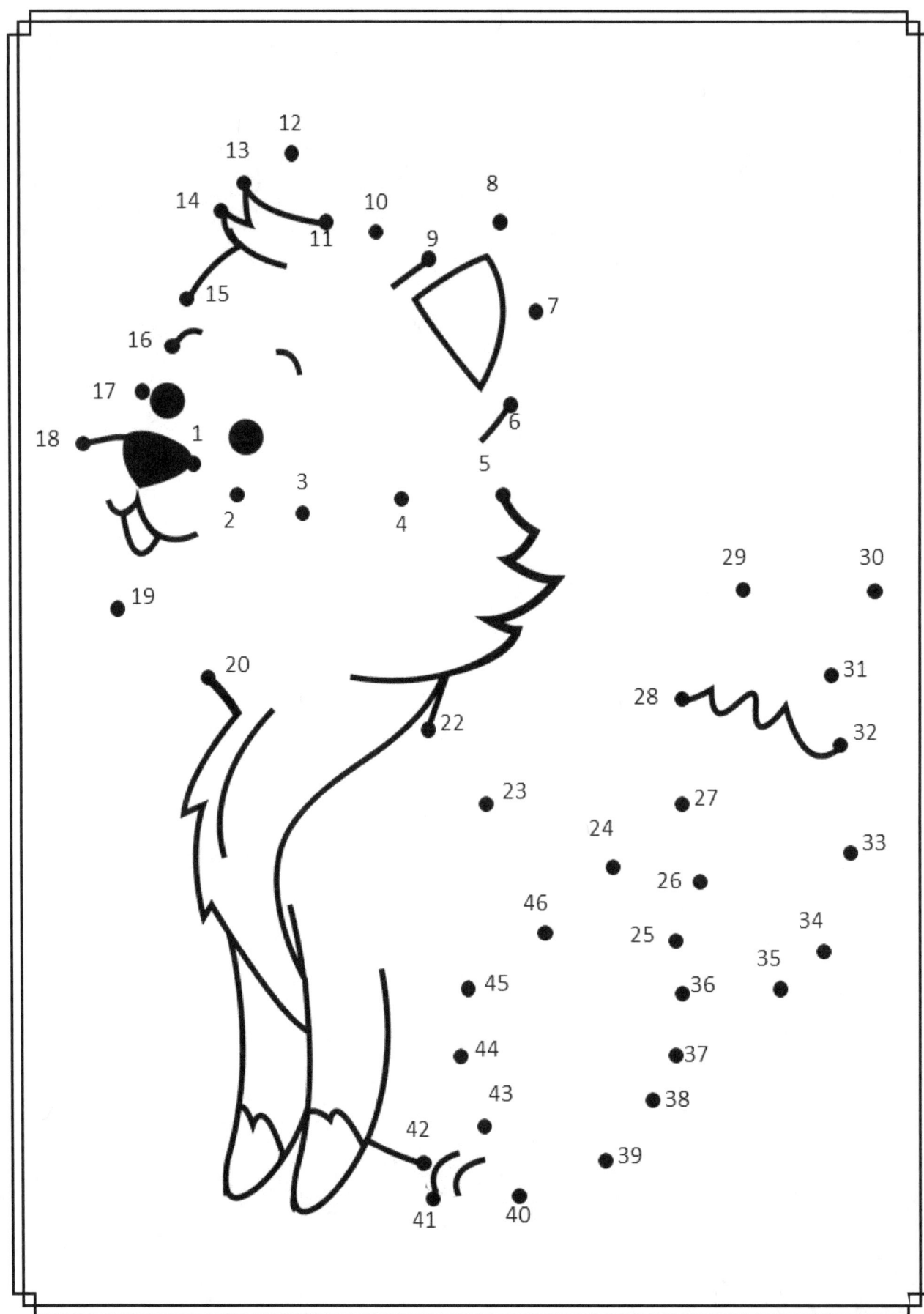

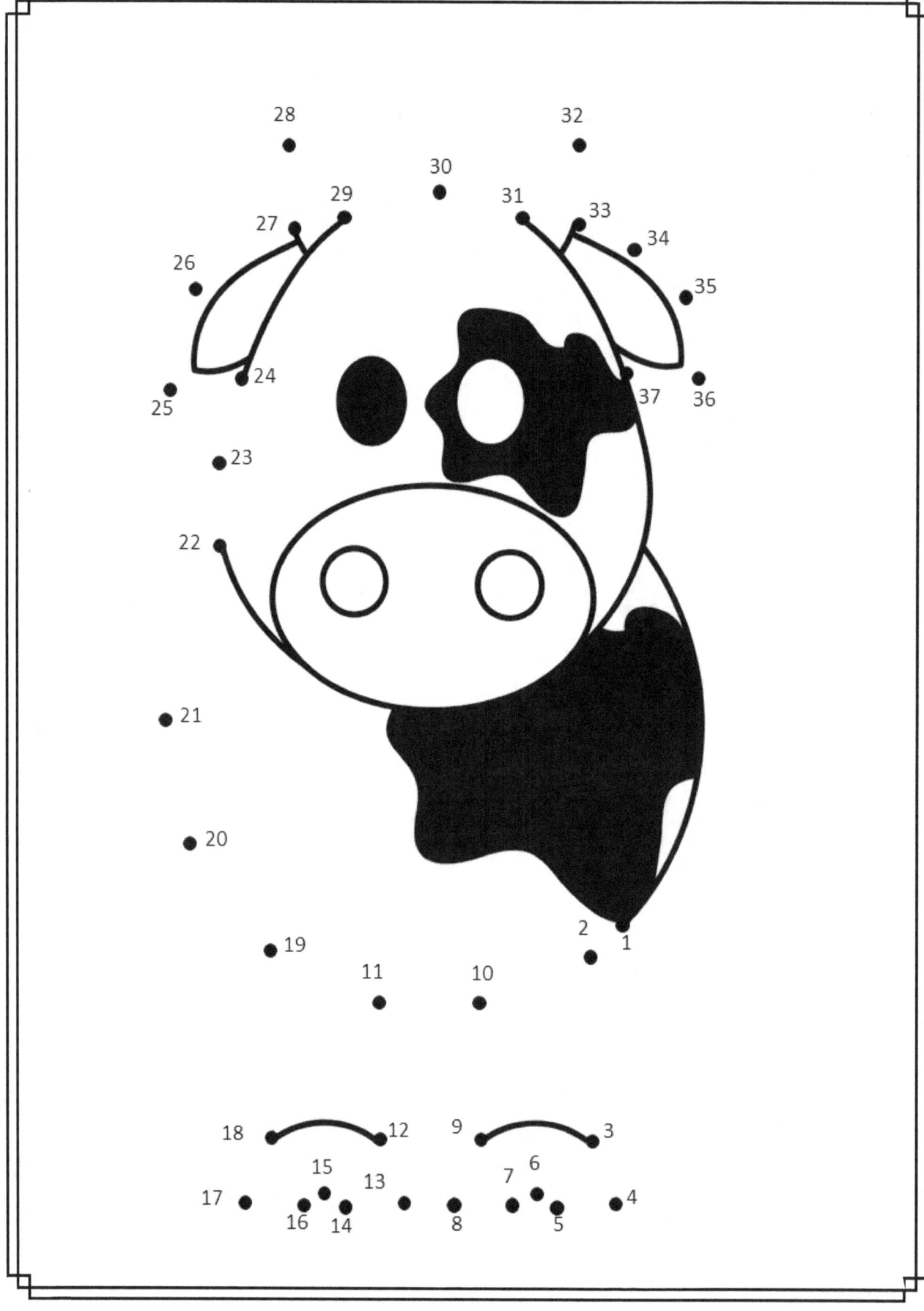

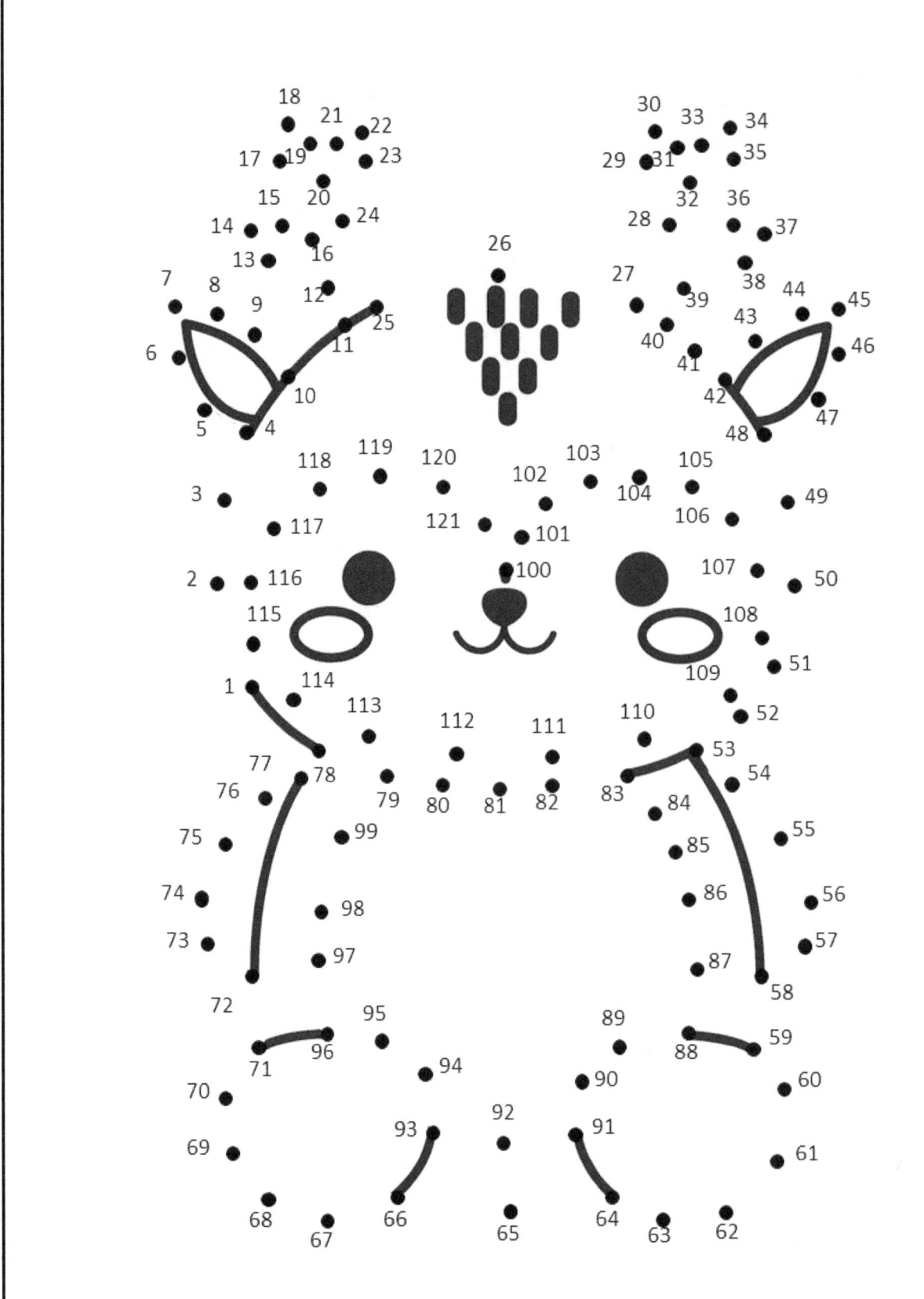

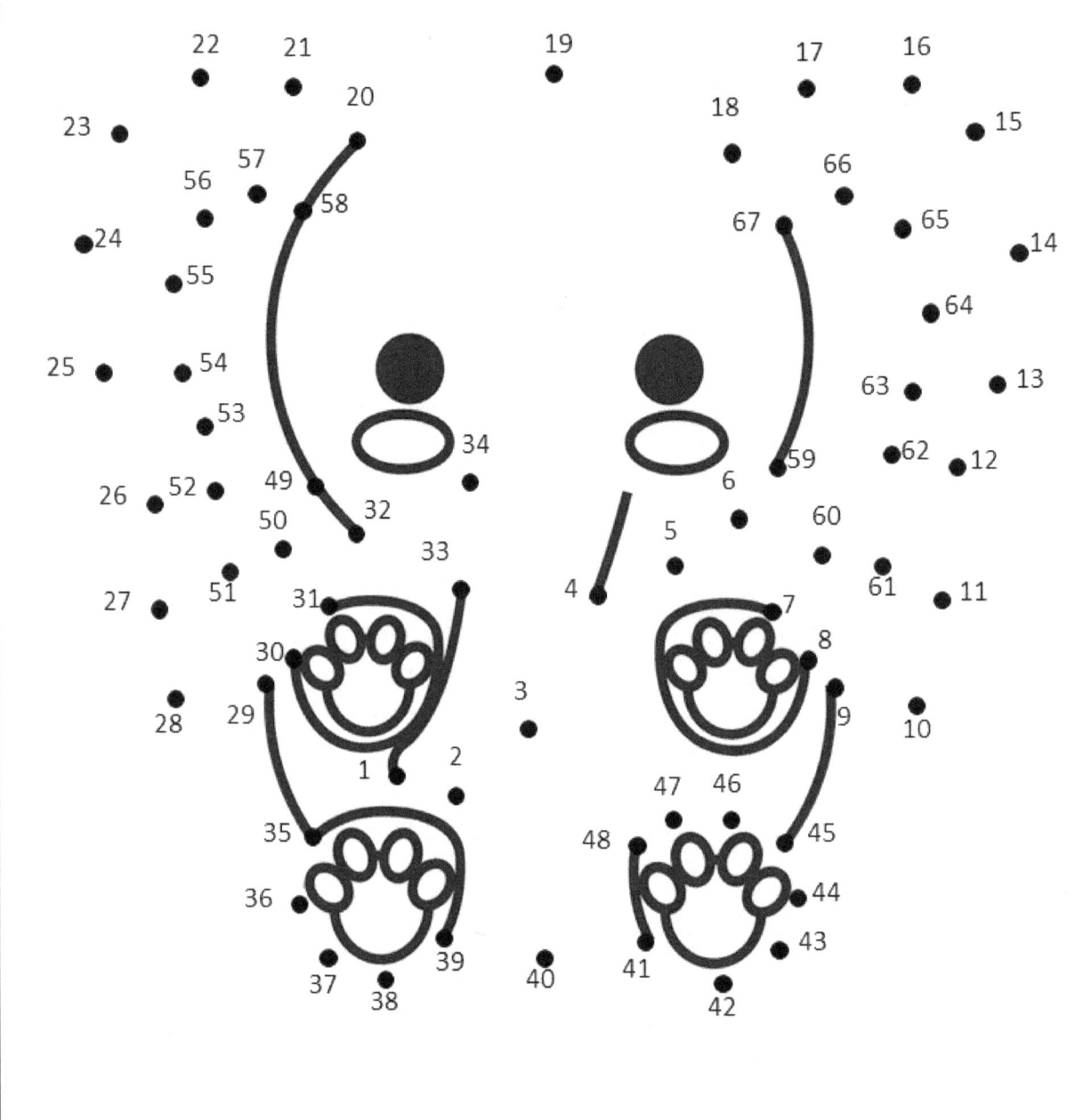

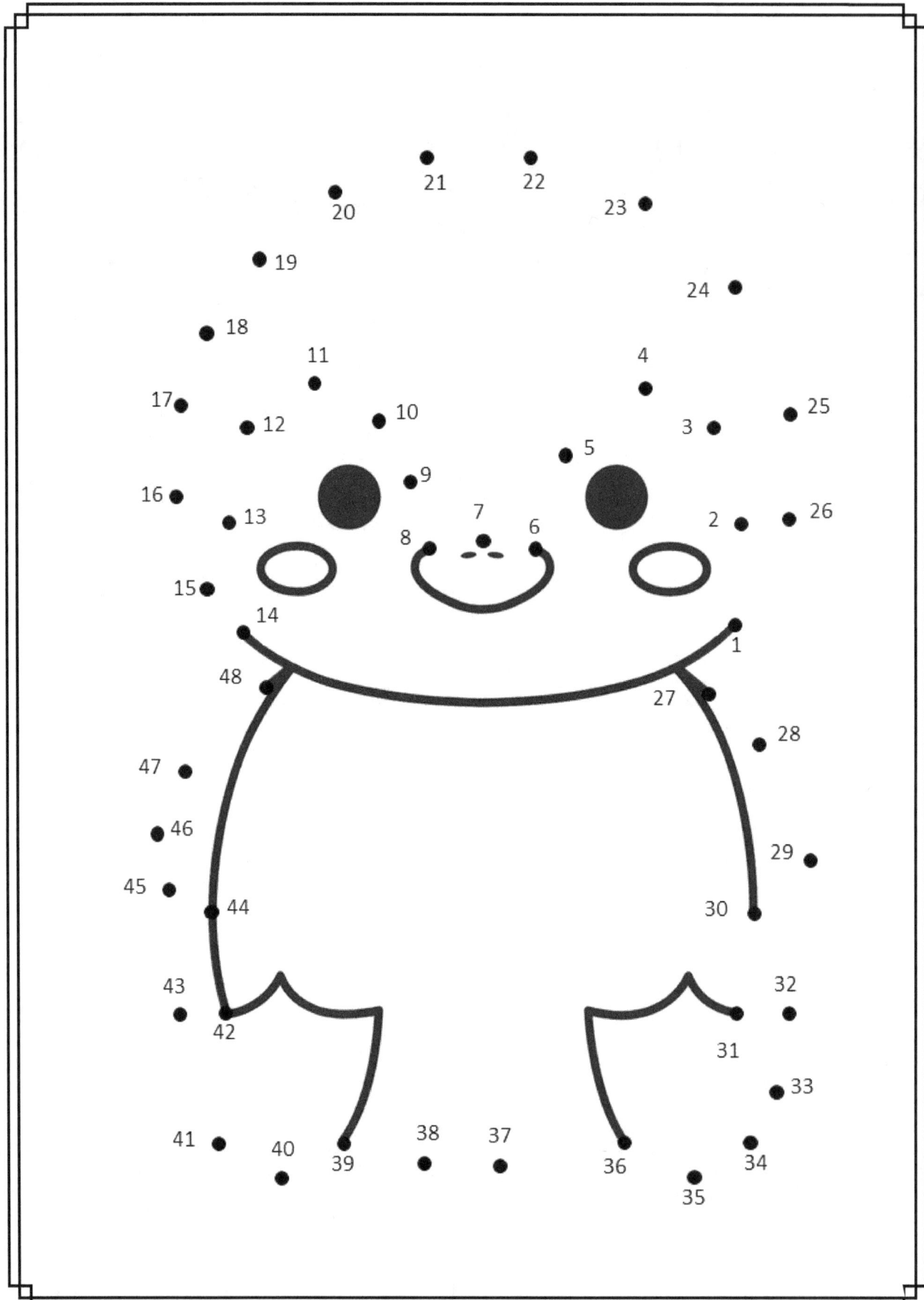

www.ingramcontent.com/pod-product-compliance
Lightning Source LLC
Chambersburg PA
CBHW082017230526
45466CB00022B/2448